MEDICAL
TRAVEL
TODAY

OPINIONS AND PERSPECTIVES ON
AN INDUSTRY IN THE MAKING

LAURA CARABELLO
Executive Editor and Publisher
Medical Travel Today

MEDICAL TRAVEL TODAY
Opinions and Perspectives on an Industry in the Making

Copyright © 2011 by Laura Carabello

ISBN 13: 978-1461147107
ISBN-10: 1461147107

Cover Design and Page Layout: Joseph Morgan
Design and Production Manager: Ervin Torres
Editor: Amanda Haar
Printing: On-Demand Publishing, LLC

Printed in the USA

CPR Strategic Marketing Communications
475 Market Street
Second Floor
Elmwood Park NJ 07407
201 641 1911
editor@medicaltraveltoday.com
www.medicaltraveltoday.com

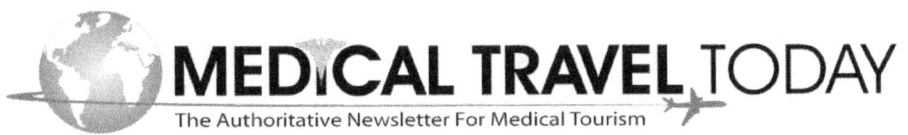

ACKNOWLEDGEMENTS

THE DEBUT of *Medical Travel Today* in 2006 fulfilled a journalism-school dream: My very own newsletter. What I never imagined was that this electronic publication would some-day reach the desktops of such a large and diverse global audience, and provide business leaders in healthcare with a platform for information exchange regarding a very nascent industry.

Even more remarkable is the fact that every day, our team receives subscription requests, along with Letters to the Editor and article submissions. Readers respond to sur-vey questions, enter drawings, express their personal opinions (or outrage!) about issues impacting medical travel, and become actively engaged in dialogue with our editorial staff as well as each other.

One of the most gratifying aspects of this journalistic endeavor is the opportunity to interview global thought leaders, and to spend a precious hour of time learning from some of the best minds in the healthcare business. It is always a treat to hear the words, "I really don't mind talking about the subject for a little longer."

The learning curve in medical travel continues, evidenced by the insights and perspectives that continually unfold during these interviews. Together with Editor Amanda Haar, we have witnessed a worldwide phenomenon: The evolution of medical travel into a globalized and integrated healthcare system.

This maturation process is still underway, and it is exciting to witness the grow-ing interest in accessing care at Centers of Excellence – wherever they are located. Qual-ity, safety and cost still govern the decision, but virtually every destination now seeks to develop both inbound and outbound medical travel volume, as well as to drive increased business among their own citizens.

To commemorate the fifth anniversary of *Medical Travel Today*, we have select-ed some of the more compelling interviews that were published. This collection not only marks five years of hard work and the dedication of resources, but it also chronicles the changing face of the industry.

Years ago as a bright-eyed newspaper reporter, I marveled at the power of the written word. Today, I am more seasoned, but still in awe of effective communications that promote innovation. My hat is off to all those who have participated in the interview pro-cess and contributed to this editorial platform.

With thanks to my husband Joseph for supporting me in this journey, to my staff at CPR Communications, and with admiration for each and every reader of *Medical Travel Today*: this compendium is a tribute to "ink on paper" and to the phenomenon of online publishing. I look forward to helping this industry grow further, and to hearing from each and every reader throughout the world.

Laura Carabello
Executive Editor and Publisher
Medical Travel Today
www.medicaltraveltoday.com
editor@medicaltraveltoday.com

CONTENTS

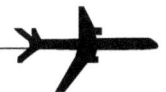

FOREWORD

WHILE THE PHENOMENOM of cross-border healthcare or "medical tourism" is hardly a new one, its growth in popularity over just the past five years has been a surprise to many media outlets – and driven by a few bold pioneers. My colleague and friend, Mrs. Laura Carabello, has the distinction of being both! Laura has clearly been on the forefront of listening to the vanguards of this space...then eloquently penning their comments and distributing them to a growing list of thousands of interested readers around the globe.

Maybe Christopher Columbus was a bit too hasty in proclaiming the earth round. Five hundred years after his discovery, we find ourselves living in a global economy. The advent of the Internet has enabled international commerce like never before. Layer social media onto this cyber platform and we are communicating with friends around the corner – and around the world – simultaneously and instantly. Clearly the world has flattened a bit since 1492!

The medical and wellness markets have enjoyed this globalization process as well. When I first explored Bumrungrad International hospital in Bangkok, Thailand in 2006, I was truly amazed at what I found. Having worked as a hospital executive for 15 years in the United States, I was convinced that my home country boasted the best care and service on earth. How myopic I was! Bumrungrad was the first Joint Commission Internationally accredited hospital in all Asia; today there are over 300 Joint Commission accredited hospitals outside of America. I have been fortunate to have surveyed 30 of them in 20 countries. Many of these facilities are built to American Institute of Arehitects (AIA) standards. They house General Electric MRIs manufactured in Florence, South Carolina, Hill-Rom beds manufactured in Indiana, Merck drugs, Stryker orthopedic implants, etc. Let's not forget the people providing the high quality care: These facilities have a plethora of U.S.-Board Certified physicians and nurses with U.S licenses. Many have information technology that prevents errors... and systems so robust that they are the envy of many Western hospital executives.

In the pages that follow, Laura Carabello shares a number of interviews that she has enjoyed with some of the disruptive innovators in this flattened world of medical tourism. She has kept her "ear to the contrail" by observing where patients are travelling to – and for which surgical procedures. You will enjoy Laura's balanced expose of this exciting emerging market!

David T. Boucher, M.P.H, FACHE, CPO
President and Chief Operating Officer
Companion Global Healthcare, Inc.
Columbia, South Carolina, USA

INTRODUCTIONS

Josef Woodman
Chief Executive Officer
Patients Beyond Borders

CONGRATULATIONS to Laura, Amanda, and everyone at CPR for helping to guide us all through five years of a relentlessly evolving medical travel marketplace. With each issue, *Medical Travel Today* helped us stay abreast of so many important topics and events: the complexities of international quality assurance, the role of telemedicine, the riddles of healthcare reform, elusive insurance players, new technologies, emerging specialties and destinations...the list goes on.

Laura's long, deep industry experience provided us perspective on how medical travel influenced (and was influenced by) so many other drivers of the larger international medical landscape—instrumentation, pharma, political and cultural opportunities and barriers, patient education, accreditation standards, and more. I particularly enjoyed the interviews, most of which originated outside the medical travel sector and brought new insight and business intelligence to our community.

Collectively, the issues of *Medical Travel Today* form a chronicle of the contemporary medical travel industry, which I believe will one day be looked upon as a catalyst for change that none of us can imagine in the moment. While it's clear that Laura shares that vision, I think she would agree with the Horace Greeley quip: "Journalism will kill you, but it will keep you alive while you're at it."

From all our staff, our sincerest appreciation for all the good work you do; we look forward to many future years of informed reading and dialog!

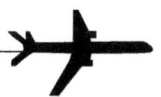

Rudy Rupak
President
Planet Hospital

I introduced Laura Carabello to medical tourism. There, I said it! And since this sentence remains in this book, Laura must believe it to be true.

However, what Laura did with it after she learned about it from me was mesmerizing. Without Laura's guidance, my company, PlanetHospital would not exist nor would it go on to dominate the consumer medical tourism space.

Looking back in all the years I've known Laura, she has been a passionate champion of medical tourism. She stuck with it, assisted in staging one of the first medical tourism conferences, and helped to spawn several industry initiatives.

Laura has become the unofficial spokesperson for medical tourism, and her persistence is nothing short of legendary. The industry accepts her bi-weekly online newsletter as the more authoritative voice than many of the pretenders to the throne.

It was only a matter of time that she would decide to publish this book, and I salute her for it. Laura will continue to shine her wonderful beacon onto this industry and will definitely contribute to its future growth.

Victor Lazzaro
Chief Executive Officer
BridgeHealth Medical

Publisher Laura Carabello, Editor Amanda Haar, and the *Medical Travel Today* team have created and built an authoritative, informative, and timely resource. I use the term resource purposefully, as it is much more than a newsletter -- it is a reliable source of information about the industry. Not only are there the insightful interviews, but also information and reporting on important conferences, presentations, and hospitals.

Case in point: Within just a few weeks in 2011, Laura Carabello was in Korea, then to Spain, and on to Costa Rica gathering updates from around the world. The in-depth interviews probe important industry issues and are broad in scope so that readers really get to know the individuals as well as the company or organizations that they represent.

Collectively, these interviews, profiles, and focused articles are a reference resource for those of us in the health care field -- not simply those involved in medical travel. News about health care conferences, major healthcare events, and key insurance points are valuable. Additionally, there has been an increased focus on the value of health care services, the combination of quality and cost as well as transparency of information. This has resulted in discussion of key providers as Centers of Excellence for their particular expertise.

The ability to report on this range of information, of course, requires a very responsible and fair presentation, and I find that this balance is always present. I may not always agree with the content or perspectives presented, and that is good. It means that views are challenged or new insights given.

All of this is becomes of interest for the HR and benefits executives, providers around the world, insurance companies and administrators, brokers and consultants, researchers, accreditation entities, and educators in this field. The newsletter reports not just on the more commonly expected international medical tourism of a U.S. resident traveling abroad, but also on intra-U.S. activities (domestic medical travel), in-bound patients to the U.S., and non U.S. citizens accessing care in various parts of the world.

In summary, *Medical Travel Today* is a must-read newsletter.

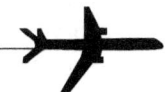

The Ethics of Medical Tourism
A U.S. Insurer Takes a Thoughtful Approach

February 2007

Special to Medical Travel Today
Introduction and Editing by Jeff Schult

It is, of course, big news in the medical tourism industry when a major media source steps up and examines what's going on, identifies the trend, moves the story forward or even just shares the experience of patients with readers or viewers.

But *Medical Travel Today* is just as fascinated - or perhaps more so - when we hear about the dialogue that's going on between professionals at high levels in managed care in the United States.

In mid July, the Harvard Pilgrim Health Care Ethics Advisory Group (EAG), in response to questions about medical tourism that percolated through the health insurance company, met to discuss medical travel from the standpoint of the ethics of the insurer. The EAG is made up of Harvard Pilgrim staff, employers, and physicians from Harvard Pilgrim's network and members. The group provides advice to Harvard Pilgrim managers and leaders on values-related aspects of issues submitted to it for consultation.

While hospitals, of course, have formal ethics panels, it is less common, even rare, for insurance companies to have such bodies. We thank Harvard Pilgrim and James E. Sabin, MD, director of the company's ethics program, for sharing with us the ethics panel's report.

The report's recommendations are strictly advisory and neither reflects current policy at Harvard Pilgrim nor predict the future. But they provide a unique glimpse into the kinds of issues managed care firms will wrestle with, as medical tourism becomes a possible or even likely option.

After describing medical tourism generally, from news reports, the report delves directly into the ethical issues. Among the conclusions:

"On the assumption that a host of important practical problems could be solved, the EAG felt that offering high quality/low cost treatment abroad could provide a win/win opportunity. If incentives were designed properly members, purchasers and HPHC could all save money while providing high quality care."

The following is excerpted from the report:

Questions for the Ethics Advisory Group
HPHC is just beginning to receive requests for treatment abroad. In the last 16 months there have been four appeals re out of country treatment - (a) to Belgium for a hip resurfacing surgical procedure that was not (at the time) FDA approved, (b) to Germany for a laparoscopic procedure for abdominal adhesions that was not FDA approved, (c) to the Philippines for a chemotherapy in a breast cancer trial for an agent that was not FDA approved or yet in trial in the U.S. and (d) to Austria for an experimental

treatment for glioblastoma multiforme (a malignant brain tumor) that was not FDA approved. Since FDA approval is typically a necessary condition for coverage all four appeals were denied.

As (a) the standard of care at overseas sites continues to improve, (b) U.S. cost escalation continues its inexorable trend, (c) marketing to potential medical tourists becomes more sophisticated and aggressive and (d) media and the web report on positive experiences with overseas treatment it is (e) inevitable that questions about medical tourism will arise with more frequency for HPHC. On July 18th the EAG was asked to offer consultation to HPHC leadership as it develops principles for future coverage policy. Questions included:

1. For enrollees with PPO products that cover out of network services and do not limit their care to a contracted network, what values considerations are relevant to defining the geographical boundaries of the PPO coverage? From the perspective of values what is the rationale for saying "yes" or "no" to overseas treatment?

2. HMO enrollees receive their care from a defined network of providers. Treatment outside of the network is ordinarily approved only if it is not available within the HMO network. What, if anything, should HPHC cover as part of its benefit structure when HMO members request outside-of-U.S. services? What values considerations are relevant to answering this question?

3. How should HPHC think about the impact of medical tourism on the host country? Suppose it appears that medical tourism is siphoning human and financial capital away from the host country system or organs for transplantation away from host country citizens on transplant waiting lists? Suppose there is suspicion that donors are being paid to provide organs?

4. It is inevitable that some HPHC members will go abroad for treatment in circumstances in which HPHC approval has been requested and denied. What values are relevant to deciding who is responsible for the cost of follow up treatment if complications occur?

Relevant Precedents

On September 21, 2000 the EAG discussed "What Level of Quality is 'Appropriate' for a Member's Care?" The case focused on a request from an HMO member for prostate cancer treatment at Johns Hopkins, based on his contention that an "appropriate" level of quality was not available within the HMO network. The report includes this paragraph:

With regard to the question of whether the relevant elements of quality have been demonstrated in an adequately objective manner the EAG made a distinction. The EAG believed that the nerve sparing technique itself had been demonstrated to be superior to non-nerve sparing surgery. It questioned, however, whether a meaningful difference between nerve sparing surgery by Dr. Walsh at Johns Hopkins and nerve sparing surgery available within the HPHC network had been objectively demonstrated. There was no doubt that Dr. Walsh is highly competent and that Mr. A strongly preferred having the surgery at Johns Hopkins with Dr. Walsh. The EAG felt, however, that it is important to distinguish between claims of superiority and objectively demonstrated superiority.

In a meeting devoted to "Developing a Framework of Values for Determining when Interventions are 'Experimental' and 'Unproven'" (November 9, 2005) the EAG reaffirmed its commitment to a high standard of evidence for coverage decisions:

The EAG emphasized that making decisions about coverage for new technologies requires a prior decision about the standards for "good enough evidence"... the EAG again strongly endorsed the high standard put forward in the Benefit Handbook[1] as consistent with the mission of "improv[ing] the health of the people we serve" and the historical medical ethics teaching - "first, do no harm."

The EAG had not deliberated about out-of-the-US treatment heretofore - July 18th involved new territory!

EAG DISCUSSION / RECOMMENDATIONS

At the outset of the discussion the EAG put the topic of medical tourism into the broad context of globalization. US healthcare occurs in a market environment and markets extend beyond national boundaries. We should expect overseas providers to compete for a share of the US health care market and US consumers to "shop" for health services abroad as well as at home. Likewise, we should expect to see outsourcing to occur in health care as it does in other industries. Already some radiologists in the HPHC network are using "nighthawk" programs in India in which US trained radiologists read scans taken at night in US facilities. And, HPHC's Perot partner has moved selected backroom functions to India. These globalizing trends will accelerate, probably quite rapidly.

The EAG recognized the many practical problems associated with treatment outside of the United States. Before HPHC considered covering overseas treatment it would need to be able to assess quality of care. The Joint Commission International certification program provides a start, and it will not be long before entrepreneurial enterprises begin to offer new quality monitoring reports. If HPHC sponsored treatment abroad it would have to ensure continuity of care for when patients returned to the US. Legal issues would have to be addressed, such as what sort of liability protections patients would have if something went wrong at a foreign hospital and whether HPHC would have any special liability in such circumstances. But the EAG conducted its deliberations on the assumption that these practical problems could be solved.

The EAG reached a strong consensus that if (a) high quality care at a favorable price was available overseas and (b) issues of continuity of care, legal liabilities, etc could be successfully addressed, then (c) covering overseas care would support many important HPHC values:

- Insofar as high quality care at a lower cost was available overseas covering it would advance the HPHC mission to "improve the health of the people we serve."
- As HPHC serves more large national accounts through its alliance with United Health it will deal increasingly with companies that have employees outside of the US and require solutions for these employees' needs. Skill in addressing overseas treatment would allow HPHC to serve its large corporate customers better.
- Self-insured companies are likely to see high quality/low cost overseas treatment for selected conditions as a benefit for themselves and their employees. In this way too, skill in addressing overseas treatment would allow HPHC to serve this segment of its corporate customers better.
- In the context of high deductible health insurance the EAG imagined that in the future health plans might wave the deductible for patients who had selected procedures done overseas. This would benefit the patients and the health plan.

5

- One EAG participant commented "the U.S. health system is clearly broken and costs are out of control...from a competitive perspective, endorsing overseas treatment would send a strong message to U.S. providers that costs must be controlled better!" Another participant commented that covering treatment abroad is a form of "outsourcing cost containment, an area managed care has largely given up on in the US!"

The EAG briefly discussed the issue of members who want to go abroad for treatment that is not FDA approved or otherwise available within the United States. The group felt that its previous recommendations with regard to a framework of values for coverage of new technologies apply to this area as well. The same standards for judging whether to cover treatment in the U.S. (FDA approval, etc) should be applied to requests for treatment overseas. Requests are likely to be more common in the future as it is easier for drug companies to do initial Phase I studies in developing countries than in the US.

With regard to the question of who should be financially responsible if members choose to go abroad for treatments for which HPHC approval has been denied the group was divided. Some felt that "health insurance covers injuries from doing dumb things like bungee jumping, so why shouldn't it cover injuries from other dumb choices, like going abroad for unapproved treatment?" Others felt that if members (a) know that their insurer does not see the requested treatment as appropriate for coverage and (b) choose to go ahead on their own then (c) they should be financially responsible for the full treatment, including (d) treatment of complications arising from the unapproved treatment.

The EAG spent the final half hour of the meeting discussing the impact of medical tourism on the host country. It recognized the possibility that high quality/ good value treatment for Americans could have negative effects on the host country:

- There could be an internal "brain drain" in the host country if the most qualified physicians gravitated towards facilities serving foreigners.
- In poor countries persons living in dire poverty may sell organs for transplant in hope of providing better for their families. The EAG debated whether individuals should be allowed to make "informed choices" about sale of organs. The consensus of the group was that even if the host country accepted voluntary sale of body parts a US health plan should govern its practices by its own values and the values reflected in the US prohibition on selling body parts.
- One participant reported having been at a presentation describing allegations that in several countries prisoners were used as a source of organs and that involuntary tissue typing was done on admission to the prison as a way of "inventorying" available organs.

The EAG recognized that HPHC cannot solve the problems of poverty in countries that host medical tourism or ensure optimal distribution of the host country's medical resources. But the group felt that the last five words of the HPHC mission - "to improve the health of the people we serve and the health of society (emphasis added)" -- should be interpreted to refer to the host country's society as well as US society. Especially for extreme examples like sale of body parts or "harvesting" transplant organs from prisoners HPHC should not serve its members by means that produce significant harms to the host country.

The EAG emphasized the importance of transparency in any developments with regard to medical tourism. Endorsing transparency means that if getting high quality treatment at a lower price is the rationale for offering coverage that should be made explicit to stakeholders. Similarly, transparency means that issues like the potential impact of medical tourism on the host country should be addressed openly and proactively. HPHC aspires to being a thought leader with regard to health care policy, and medical tourism offers an opportunity to speak out in an educational manner.

Summary
1. On the assumption that a host of important practical problems could be solved, the EAG felt that offering high quality/low cost treatment abroad could provide a win/win opportunity. If incentives were designed properly members, purchasers and HPHC could all save money while providing high quality care.
2. The EAG felt that the same values framework HPHC uses for deciding about coverage for treatments in the US (FDA approval, evidence base, etc) should be applied to requests for treatments abroad.
3. The issue of how medical tourism impacts host countries is complex, but the EAG felt that these impacts should be considered if and when HPHC considers coverage of overseas treatments. The EAG felt that fundamental HPHC and U.S. values - such as the view that body parts should not be sold (or, in the case of prisoners, taken) - should be adhered to, even if the host country accepts these practices.
4. The EAG strongly supported the active way in which (the referring manager) and his colleagues were addressing medical tourism - beginning to plan for the area in a proactive manner, not simply responding to trends as they emerged. The group thanked (the manager) and his colleagues for allowing it to undertake this anticipatory ethical analysis of the area before any problems hit the fan!

Editor's Note: *Harvard Pilgrim's website is:* www.harvardpilgrim.org. *Dr. James Sabin has launched a blog on the ethics of healthcare organizations at:* http://healthcare-organizationalethics.blogspot.com.

[1] The section on exclusions in the Harvard Pilgrim Schedule of Benefits states "Drugs, devices, treatments or procedures which are Experimental or Unproven [are excluded from coverage]." Here is how the HPHC Benefit Handbook defines the key terms:

A service, procedure, device or drug will be deemed Experimental or Unproven by HPHC under this Member Agreement for use in the diagnosis or treatment of a particular medical condition if any of the following is true:

- *The service, device or drug is not recognized in accordance with generally accepted medical standards as being safe and effective for the use in the evaluation or treatment of the condition in question. In determining whether a service has been recognized as safe or effective in accordance with generally accepted medical standards, primary reliance will be placed upon data from published reports in authoritative medical or scientific publications that are subject to peer review by qualified medical or scientific experts prior to publication. In the absence of any such reports, it will generally be determined that a service, procedure, device or drug is not safe and effective for the use in question.*
- *In the case of a drug, the drug has not been approved by the United States Food and Drug Administration (FDA) (This does not include off-label use of FDA approved drugs).*

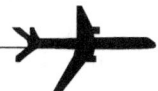

Electronic Health Records and Medical Tourism

March 2007

By Laura Carabello and Jeff Schult

The world is closer to the grail of universal Electronic Health Records (EHRs) than most people think, and continued progress will help to make medical travel safer, according to one of the leading innovators in medical informatics, David C. Kibbe, M.D., MBA.

Dr. Kibbe is a senior adviser to the Center for Health Information Technology (HIT) of the American Academy of Family Physicians (AAFP) and a principal of The Kibbe Group LLC in Pittsboro, North Carolina. He is co-developer of the ASTM Continuity of Care Record (CCR).

"The 'Pie in the Sky' is that, ultimately, most providers and institutions would have EHR infrastructure and a paperless environment," he said in an interview with Medical Travel Today. "We're seeing it occur in the United States rather rapidly, under adverse circumstances. In Minnesota, 67 percent of institutions are now using EHR, a statistic that might surprise a lot of people. The top-flight medical destinations pretty much all have EHR."

Going forward, Kibbe said, medical records technology must provide for:

"… Secure, private, and accurate aggregation and transport of all relevant personal health information, using tested international standards and methods, to assure that patients' experience continuity of information flow between their medical home and medical tourism providers and institutions, and are assured that nothing important about their medical history gets left behind."

He expects EHR and CCR standards to evolve in several ways, on different fronts. "Global destination parties" such as Microsoft (the recently opened-for-business Healthvault.com) and Google (still in demo mode) have already launched online health record initiatives. Another likelihood is that some group with international credibility will step in and provide guidance and standards; and yet a third probability is that a business association, an industry consortium or even an individual business with proprietary but advanced technology will take the lead.

Dr. Kibbe views universal EHR/CCR as inevitable, given the likely improvement in quality of care, reduction of errors and cost savings.

"There is too much of an incentive to succeed," he said. Problems between countries such as language will be resolved by electronic translation and/or settling on English as the common language for EHRs, he said.

Besides his work in EHRs/CCRs, Dr. Kibbe is also an experienced clinician who practiced medicine in private and academic settings for more than 15 years, while also teaching informatics at the School of Public Health, University of North Carolina at Chapel Hill, and founded two medical software companies. In 2005, readers of the magazine *Modern Physician* voted him one of the 50 Most Powerful Physician Executives in Healthcare.

From 2002 until 2006, Dr. Kibbe was the founding director of the Center for Health Information Technology for the AAFP, the membership organization that represents over 95,000 U.S. family doctors. The Center is now the locus of the AAFP's technical expertise, advocacy, and research and member services associated with HIT, and a leading national resource on information and communications technology for physicians.

During Dr. Kibbe's tenure as Director of the Center for HIT, AAFP physician member adoption and use of EHRs more than tripled, from 12 percent to over 40 percent.

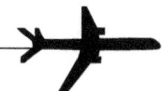

Linda Ludwick
President
Health Care Administrators Association
"The Future of Medical Tourism and TPAs"

April 2007

The enormous amount of recent press dedicated to the subject of medical tourism has caught the attention of consumers and Third Party Administrators (TPAs) alike. In a recent conversation with Linda Ludwick, president of the Health Care Administrators Association (HCAA) and executive director of Mountain States Administrative Services, *Medical Travel Today* learned that more and more TPAs are looking seriously at how medical tourism may shape their future offerings.

"Without a doubt, brokers and TPAs are looking hard at medical tourism as an opportunity. In the last year alone, our top five clients have begun looking earnestly at how they might incorporate medical tourism into their offerings," says Ludwick. Among the questions being asked are:

- Should we offer it?
- What type of cost savings could we see?
- What's the associated liability?
- What's the quality of the site and the provider?
- How do we implement a medical tourism offering?
- Should we implement this ourselves or partner with others?

According to Ludwick, TPAs aren't the only ones asking questions. "At a recent employee meeting with a client of Mountain States, an employee stood up and asked how soon the company would begin offering a medical tourism benefit. That was a first for me, but I expect we'll see more and more of it in the near future."

In order to help TPAs better understand exactly what medical tourism is all about, the HCAAs annual TPA University to be held July 16-18 in San Francisco will feature panel discussions on the subject of medical tourism.

"We feel that medical tourism is one of the key issues for TPAs today. We're all engaged in a constant struggle to compete with the BUCAs (the Blues, United, Cigna, and Aetna) – all of whom are currently offering or about to offer medical tourism benefits," says Ludwick. "If we as TPAs don't offer it, we'll lose our competitive edge."

For more information on the HCAA and the TPA University, visit:
http://hcaa.org/tpauniversity.html.

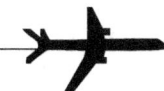

David T. Boucher, M.P.H., FACHE, CPO
President & Chief Operating Officer
Companion Global Healthcare, Inc.

July 2007

Editor's Note: *At the time of this interview, David Boucher was the assistant vice president for health care services at BlueCross BlueShield of South Carolina. In this capacity, he was administratively responsible for Companion Global Healthcare, commercial EDI transactions and provider e-commerce, provider education, the inquiry response center, complementary and alternative health programs and medical management services. In the past few years, Boucher has been quoted in more than 200 national health care publications, as well as on NBC Nightly News. Medical Travel Today caught up with Boucher in late July for a lengthy telephone chat. The following is Part One of the interview.*

Medical Travel Today **(MTT): Hi David. Welcome to** *Medical Travel Today*, **and thanks for talking with us and our readers. We've been following the news about Companion Global Healthcare (a new subsidiary of BlueCross BlueShield of South Carolina) ever since you announced your medical tourism initiative in February. In a way, we've been waiting for you. For a while, it has seemed like just a matter of time before larger corporate healthcare entities in the U.S. became involved in medical tourism. You're sort of "first in," and moving fast. I wonder if you could give me a sense of some of the history and process that led BlueCross BlueShield of South Carolina to this point. Where did you begin?**

David Boucher (DB): I guess on a couple of fronts… By way of background I'm an ex-hospital CEO. I've worked with Quorum Health Resources and Quorum Health Group hospitals for about 15 years. So I've been on the provider side for a fairly significant amount of time and I was the CEO of hospitals in both North and South Carolina.

Currently and for the last several years with BlueCross of South Carolina, I directed our medical management programs for utilization management, disease management, complex care management … also provider satisfaction and Web technology on the provider side for commercial business. One of the other areas I also direct are our complementary and alternative medicine programs, where we've been the leader amongst the Blues in the whole area of value added programs.

We pre-negotiated discount programs with organizations like Belltone, TLC Vision, American Cosmetic Surgery Networks, companies like that, because we know that increasing numbers of our members and Americans in general are going outside of their standard benefit plans for various things that are health and wellness related.

So we've been fairly aggressive about that. Our members can show their ID card and they receive fairly significant discounts from our partners, and also have access to both discounts and various pre-priced procedures. So that's one of the areas I manage.

Fast forward: I'd been picking up in the popular media about this whole trend of medical tourism from the news in Business Week, on 60 Minutes, etc. So I reached out to a couple of colleagues who dabble in international healthcare and I said, "Look, my wife and I are thinking about traveling to someplace exotic to check out this emerging trend ... so we asked around and, independently, two or three of them said: 'If you are going to make a trip, go to the medical tourism leader in the world, Bumrungrad International. That's where you really want to go.'

I was thinking about the Philippines or South America or really any place, it was just that we decided we were going to do something different. So I reached out and struck up first e-mail and then a phone conversation with Mack Banner, the CEO of Bumrungrad. Mack and I both worked for Quorum at the same time. He was at a Quorum facility in California at the same time I was a CEO at a facility in North Carolina. So we talked and he said, "Come on over, we'd like to show you around."

So last June 30 (2006) we got on a plane and flew to Bangkok. Neither of us had been to Southeast Asia ... and what I ended up doing there, basically, was a fairly intense, yet unofficial, hospital survey. Not the identical way the Joint Commission does ... though I had participated in a number of JCAHO surveys here in the U.S. But I was pretty rigorous.

So we stayed at Bumrungrad Suites--the hospital-owned hotel--about 50 yards from the facility. We were greeted at the airport 10:30-11:00 at night by the same concierge folks that greet other Bumrungrad medical tourists ... I had asked Mack really not to do anything differently than they would when they greeted medical tourists. So we stayed at the Suites and walked back and forth to the hospital and spent a good part of our time from Friday morning through the following Tuesday evening with the hospital staff. That was pretty much my "vacation." I gowned up and went into the operating rooms, recovery rooms, central linen, central sterile supply, dietary, you name it and I was there. I spent a full day with Dr. Peter Morley, the medical director; The Bumrungrad staff was very forthcoming with quality and patient satisfaction information. I was thoroughly impressed; I had never seen a hospital like that. And when you combine the quality with the hospitality level that they can afford to provide, and that the Thais enjoy proffering... well, my wife and I were just blown away with the whole experience.

When we had just boarded our departure flight at the Charlotte Airport, I remember telling my wife: "I think that this may be a life-changing experience. I have no idea what that means, but, I just think that we're really going to learn and do some really interesting things." And, as we were boarding our return flight in Bangkok, my wife said, without me even prompting her: "If myself or anybody in my family needs an operation and we can withstand a 25-hour flight, we're coming to Bumrungrad."

That was it for me; the marketing was done. My wife said that without the understanding that women make a majority of the healthcare decisions for their family. If she could make that call, so would a lot of other women, for their families. We're true blue Americans -- my son is a Marine in Iraq right now, and so it was not about trashing U.S. healthcare or anything like that.

We live here in South Carolina. We did not know really what to expect over there, Jeff. We were just incredibly surprised by what we found.

MTT: It sounds like we've had some similar experiences. When I went overseas for dental work I was a little nervous and concerned and I came back as an evangelist for it in some ways. I didn't write my book as a proselytizer -- I tried to write it objectively -- but I certainly had a life-changing experience.

DB: That was the experience we had, absolutely. When I returned from Bangkok I had the opportunity to talk to some of the senior staff at BlueCross BlueShield of South Carolina. We tend to seek out Blue Ocean instead of fighting out in the marketplace, fighting over the same fixed customer base. We're always looking to see how we can expand the base -- how we can make markets. So that was how we started to look at the whole globalization of healthcare -- we began to enumerate benefits that really offered the opportunity to create a market.

So--fast forward to the beginning of this year--we are, as all Blue plans are, an independent licensee of the Blue Cross Association and we are prevented from contracting with out-of-state hospitals ... and obviously, Bangkok and Singapore and other places are out of state. So we formed a company, Companion Global Healthcare Inc., as a subsidiary for what we are doing in this area ... and we'll give it several years and see where it goes. We own and operate Companion Life Insurance Co. and we have had, for over twenty years, the Companion Property and Casualty Co. The Companion name is at the top of our building.

MTT: So you've got some branding on that already.
DB: You bet. We've owned several "Companion" companies over the years, so we have a little bit of leverage there. So what we've done now is we've partnered with World Access. (World Access, a member of the global Mondial Assistance Group, is a leading provider of travel insurance, international healthcare, and assistance products.)

World Access provides travel agency services, case management services for those patients interested in traveling abroad, and they will coordinate with the provider care community to get the member there as quickly as reasonably possible and make sure they can get good care. They have a contracted network of air ambulances at their fingertips as well.

That, we felt, offered several advantages -- World Access is a known entity amongst the commercial insurance and business world. We really felt like they would do a great job, being part of one of the biggest companies in the world. They have their own travel agency. We could have partnered locally but these folks ... well, for example, if they have a patient who is seeking to travel to have a knee replaced, who can't afford a business or first class ticket to Thailand, what they will try to do is work with the member and say "If you can delay your trip by one day, we can get you bulkhead seating on all legs of your flight" ... they would naturally think in those terms, in terms of working with the customer as a patient.

MTT: I was curious about the relationship with Companion Global and how you were doing this because I talked to a lot of the people who have gotten into this as a business. And it is apparent that these companies have to start creating some value and start figuring out how to scale what they do, because when the Blues get into this they're not going to be doing it for 100 people a year. They're going to scale it up and perhaps blow the little companies out of the water.
DB: Of course, that's critical, being able to scale ... our parent company manages call centers and large claims operations. These are some of our core competencies.

But we really felt like in the early offing we would subcontract out to people (World Access) who really knew what they were doing in International travel markets and not try to replicate it.

Editors Note: Medical Travel Today *caught up with Boucher in late July 2007 for a lengthy telephone chat. The following is Part Two of the interview.*

Medical Travel Today (MTT): One of the questions I had, you almost answered (in Part 1) and it surprised me a little. I was going to ask what obstacles you had overcome internally? I assume there were some objections and it sounds like from the top down you guys "got it."
David Boucher (DB): Absolutely, we really have. And I think the NBC piece (NBC News, May 15, 2007) helped a bit. NBC interviewed me, and indicated that we are one of the first companies to get involved in this … so that really helped to confirm that we were on the right track. So there weren't really any internal barriers. It's just that when you try to explain, "Here's where this thing may go …" … well, certainly, I get a few people raising eyebrows, saying, "Bangkok, Thailand? Singapore? Seoul?"

MTT: Like, what are you, crazy?
DB: Exactly. They may not come out and say it -- because I think I have a pretty decent track record for making things work outside the box -- but we'll see. What we're doing now, Jeff, is our 1.5 million members have access to these options, for Bumrungrad … as an affinity program. There are enough other folks that have gone out and started services for which they're trying their best to get covered members to do this, to go overseas. We have attempted just the opposite -- leveraging an existing membership base.

MTT: How does it work as a value-add for the patient? Why would a patient choose it?
DB: They wouldn't. First, personally, we know a number of folks around the country -- the estimates are 600,000 to a million people last year -- have elected to go abroad for surgery. If you just pro-rate the numbers of the 80,000 American patients that received services at Bumrungrad last year, about 1,200 were from South Carolina, just based on population estimates. So right off the top … the question is, why would a member for any commercial payer or TPA with a $250 or $500 deductible spend $1,500 for a plane ticket just to go to Bumrungrad for care?

Well they probably wouldn't. But we needed to go through this first step of what we consider an iterative process for a few reasons, primarily to raise member awareness. We are surprised at the amount of press that this has received and that helps to raise consumer awareness as well … but also, it has helped us to open dialogue with staff from various payers who actually shape benefit structure. We have had requests from multiple human resource brokers, companies that work with different employer groups

MTT: I get calls from New York companies whose names you would recognize and they just want me to tell them what's going on…
DB: That's how this trend will continue to gain momentum. . Here's an example, the CEO of a prospective group hears about Companion Global Healthcare and medical tourism on National Public Radio back in February and begins to ponder the financial impact of waiving the $2,000 deductible in his employee's medical plan if they choose to receive expensive surgical services at Bumrungrad. So that was great, and there are ways to do that and make it attractive or compelling.

That's where medical travel is going --small steps are getting our organization to where we're envisioning we would be between now and the January 1 benefit cycle.

MTT: It sounds like the market and the demand shape what you offer.
DB: Exactly, we need to be market-driven….and we're starting to have groups ask questions. We began advertising in a few media outlets, notably United Airlines' Hemisphere magazine. So we have begun to strategically position a few ads which focus on both patients and HR directors.

MTT: So you guys haven't sent a patient yourself?
DB: Correct.

MTT: I just wanted to make sure. I was pretty sure that was the case. That did kind of amuse me as far as a lot of the press went. "OK, are they actually doing this yet?" Yet I think it's a very big thing and I think it's a tipping point for medical tourism.
DB: You bet. We're neither surprised nor discouraged about the limited patient traffic thus far. But remember that our website (www.CompanionGlobalHealthcare.com) has received over 200,000 hits now in just about five months.

MTT: I think it's interesting the way you're rolling it out.
DB: We're just starting to do some advertising now. And I've spent a little bit of time this week developing a plan focused on stimulating specific patient interest. We have spent much of our organization's early life been building infrastructure – we're only 3 ½ months old. So we're trying to follow up on every single market lead if we can.

MTT: You're doing a good job of answering all my questions before I ask them. Have international hospitals been ringing your phone? Have you gotten that kind of reaction?
DB: Yes they have. Off the hook.

MTT: I thought so.
DB: I've been on the phone a lot. I went to visit a couple of hospitals in Mexico back in January and we don't intend to forge a relationship there at this point. I went to see a hospital in England back in April and, just because of logistics, it's not going to work either. But we are actively in the process of evaluating other facilities in overseas locales…and we are being selective in terms of quality and hospitality services.

Although we are aggressive in seeking other opportunities we are also conservative when it comes to risk. Many critics of medical travel suggest that it's only going to take one or two maladventures in this business to arrest the trend. And that could happen even with the best hospitals and care. Every patient responds to anesthesia differently. We want to be able to mitigate that risk as much as we can.

MTT: I've heard it suggested in the media that other insurers and HMOs and the like are looking very closely at medical tourism and that some of them will be following suit very soon. Would you care to venture some speculation on that?
DB: Not really -- it's hard to tell. Healthcare is a local phenomenon and it's hard to know what's going on in other states.

MTT: When people ask me, "Is this going to happen?" I tend to say, well, certainly based on the cost differential and the reputation for quality, U.S. companies and organizations have an obligation to shareholders and workers to look at it as an option.

DB: You bet, and that's what I think. I've heard…that some of the senior staff at other commercial payers recently visited Bumrungrad and other high-quality international hospitals. The popular media has helped this whole process, and again, it has come from sources with pretty good reputations like 60 Minutes, Good Morning America, *Newsweek, The Economist*…they've all run pieces.

MTT: Some of the media have really educated themselves. If you looked at stories about this 4 or 5 years ago, it was all about crazy people going overseas. I think it was 2004-05 when some media people starting looking at this and figured out it was for real.

DB: And I think it's just a matter time before any company in a margin-sensitive sector says, "We're going to take a look into this; we're going to put a global surgical option into our benefit plan and we'll see where it goes."

MTT: One other question -- do you deal JCI accreditation as a prerequisite for overseas hospitals as far as the American market?

DB: We're only going to contemplate JCI accreditation within network. Part of the reason is that a certain percentage of American consumers recognize the Joint Commission as a trusted stamp of approval, that's number one; number two is that there's an increased comfort level that the Joint Commission has been involved in giving the medical staff and the hospital's credentialing process their blessing. I recall as a hospital CEO the whole healthcare credentialing process is something the Joint Commission takes very seriously and we are comforted by that.

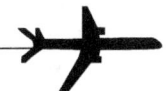

Matthew Haddad
Founder & Chief Executive Officer
Medversant Technologies, LLC

January 2008

*Patient safety continues to be one of the top concerns for consumers considering travel-
ing abroad for medical care. At this time, there is no single repository of information
on the licensing and status of providers in the various countries offering care to medical
tourists.*

*One individual who has been giving this fact some serious thought and con-
sideration is Matthew Haddad, founder and CEO of Medversant Technologies, LLC, the
leading provider of web-based health care practitioner management applications. The
company's Encompass TM technology is used across the country by hospital systems and
managed care organizations to continuously monitor the status of their affiliated providers, thus increasing patient safety and reducing liability.*

Medical Travel Today *recently had the opportunity to talk with Matt about
how the systems and technology his company implements might be applied to medical
tourism in both the near and distant future. What follows is an excerpt from that conversation.*

***Medical Travel Today* (MTT): First, tell us a bit about how you got involved
in the data management side of health care.**
Matthew Haddad (MH): Certainly. I actually began my professional life as an attorney, mostly for commercial finance and mergers and acquisitions. I then had the
opportunity to become part of a start-up involving home infusion therapy systems. In
that business, you're essentially operating a hospital without walls and that exposed
me to the healthcare industry in a big way. I was working with providers, hospitals,
pharmaceutical companies, insurers, patients… you name it. One thing that was very
apparent to me was that the technology systems for healthcare were very challenged.
There simply was no such thing as real-time information.

From that company, I moved on to buy a web-based medical billing company.
I realized fairly quickly that billing was not where I wanted to be. The constraints of
HIPAA made it difficult to create a shared platform that would be accepted by health-
care organizations.

The area of provider credentialing, however, seemed to have promise. While
traditionally overlooked and neglected, credentialing was one of the most important
processes that directly affected patient safety. Credentialing protects patients from
unlicensed, sanctioned or otherwise unqualified providers.

The process was terribly inefficient. Providers constantly had to send the
same extensive background information to numerous organizations over and over.
These organizations, in turn, took it upon themselves to verify all this information
manually, resulting in departments that seemed like one big sea of paper files and
sticky notes. The chances of error or of the work just not getting done were high.
This was a perfect example of an administrative process that could be streamlined by

an automated, web-based application. This would improve information flow, increase efficiencies on all fronts, and enhance patient safety…it was perfect. From all that, Medversant was founded.

MTT: Tell us a bit about the types of clients you work with and the services you provide.
MH: We currently have clients in every state and Puerto Rico. We work with virtually any organization that's involved in credentialing. Those include big insurance companies, hospital systems, surgery centers, nursing homes, dialysis companies, home health, imaging… you name it. What we do is provide continuous monitoring of their employees' licensure and other credentials.

In the simplest terms, we access the information in a number of databases and run it against our clients' files, warning of issues as they arise and providing real time updates. The information is all out there. We just simplify the match and merge process.

MTT: What opportunities do you see in the world of medical tourism?
MH: Medical tourism is hugely exciting. The cost benefits are obvious on many levels. Plus, I see the industry as an opportunity to increase the quality of care globally, particularly since there are many skillful practitioners around the world who could potentially be accessed.

To ensure that the industry realizes its potential, we must create credentialing standards and a connected repository for all relevant information. Consumers want to feel comfortable making health care choices, especially when it involves traveling abroad. A systemized, centralized and accessible credentials record would help provide that comfort. Plus, current technology can ensure that consumers are able to access that information with ease.

Presently, consumers can access only very limited information about their providers in the US, but they may be able to obtain much more provider information internationally, because there are often fewer, if any, cultural and legal barriers to allowing access in other countries. This difference could ultimately benefit us all in terms of ability to vet our own providers.

MTT: How feasible is the idea of establishing a common set of health care standards globally?
MH: Having a universal set of health care standards is a very realistic goal. We already have a precedent for that in the existing standards of international organizations such as the World Health Organization and the Joint Commission International. To take that further is just a matter of agreeing upon standards for our providers and facilities, then performing the credentialing to ensure that those standards are met. Countries that really want to grow as a medical tourism destination can help themselves by modernizing access to provider data through cost effective technology solutions such as Medversant's.

MTT: What about the technology end of things? Will that translate?
MH: Sure. You could use the same methodology around the world as in the US. It's just a matter of linking up to different existing databases or perhaps even creating new ones. We currently do credentials verification for many foreign providers who provide care here in the U.S. It works.

MTT: Matt, thank you for your time and for sharing your vision for the future of medical tourism and global care.

To learn more about Medversant, visit www.medversant.com. *Matt Haddad can be reached at* mhaddad@medversant.com.

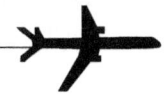

Barbara Cox
Senior Principal & Service Line Leader

John Vitalis
Senior Principal
Noblis Center for Health Innovation

January 2008

When the Noblis Center for Health Innovation (www.noblis.org/healthcare), a highly regarded organization that assists both public and private sector organizations achieve their missions through strategy, facility planning, information management and performance innovation, released its list of forecast trends for healthcare, we here at Medical Travel Today *were excited to see medical tourism on the list.*

We contacted John Vitalis, a Senior Principal at Noblis, and his colleague Barbara Cox, a Senior Principal and Service Line Leader for information management, and asked if they might be willing to talk with us about what specifically drove them to include the industry on their list for the first time — and what they see for the future.

They graciously accepted and offered the following observations about what the future might hold for consumers, clinicians, and businesses involved in the field.

Medical Travel Today (MTT): We're obviously very excited to know that our industry has caught your attention and that you see it to potentially have great influence on management and delivery in the future. Can you tell us specifically what factors prompted you to include it on your trends list?
John Vitalis (JV): There were really three main reasons for its inclusion on our list. First was the growth of the industry. We've observed a significant increase in growth, particularly in the number of US citizens traveling abroad for care.
Barbara Cox (BC): Yes, and the sheer number of sales people we're running into at conferences and in healthcare facilities who are actively recruiting patients to travel abroad is something we've never seen before.

The whole notion of travel abroad for healthcare has become so widely accepted that you'll even see a box on customs slips asking you if your reason for travel involved medical care.
JV: That's right. The second reason is the number of prestigious healthcare organizations that have established a position in the marketplace or are seeking to do so, is really noteworthy. We're talking about really prestigious providers such as Duke, Johns Hopkins, and Harvard Medical International. Each is seeking to find a way to operate in the emerging international arena.
BC: We're seeing proposals coming in the door quite regularly for various things from planning facilities abroad, to finding new ways in which they might handle their process side to allow for more international care relationships. Plus, there's the whole technical side of things. Organizations are asking what they need to do in order to communicate effectively across borders. And that communication goes beyond data

sharing to overcoming cultural differences about how you communicate, when you communicate, and what's appropriate to share.

The whole way these organizations are looking at international healthcare has shifted dramatically. In the eighties, organizations sought out people from abroad to come to the US for care. Now it's about establishing entities in those other countries to provide care. Some of this will be accomplished by building facilities, some through partnerships or contracted facility management, or by providing clinicians.

JV: The third thing is the number of very important issues that must be considered by both the organizations and patients as they consider embarking on international healthcare.

MTT: Going back to your second point, regarding the various organizations looking for ways to grow in the market, it sounds like companies are going about it in many different ways. Have you seen one way that's proving particularly effective?

BC: No, not really. How an organization goes about embarking on this type of international growth is largely dependent upon the culture of the organization, where they are in maturity in terms of handling international relationships, and where they want to be in the long run.

MTT: Turning back to look at the United States, how is medical tourism changing the face of American healthcare in the future?

JV: Based upon what we've seen in terms of trends and data, medical tourism will definitely continue to grow. The reasons are plentiful — the rising cost of healthcare, growing market opportunities internationally, opportunities to expand the footprint, and more employer interest -- particularly on the part of small employers. Also, as more people engage in it and share their experiences and money savings, others will begin to see it as a viable alternative to care.

BC: I agree. The truth is, competition drives healthcare. The interest from different organizations toward cost will increase competition. US providers are going to have to take a long hard look at how they are providing services.

As for health plans, they are definitely looking to offer different services. They're going to start offering different products that include medical tourism. Some may even provide incentives to members based upon cost reduction. It may be in the form of a rebate or a discount or something else, but they're definitely looking for ways to push members in that direction.

MTT: Do you see care on the local level being affected?

JV: Most providers won't be directly impacted. Most simply don't see themselves as competing globally. They're more concerned about competing with the hospital across town. The major academic centers will be the ones most concerned. They're the ones already operating in that arena and with market share to lose.

It's possible some local providers might find themselves losing referrals if they're in a market with organizations that practice globally. Patients, payers and employers are going to be looking for alternatives and they might feel that to some degree.

BC: The major players who will be focusing globally will be working with their providers – they may even transplant doctors across the globe to ensure a standard of care is adopted across the world under their umbrella.

MTT: Let's talk about those organizations that will be seeking to operate internationally. What are the kinds of things that they'll need to be alert to or sensitive to consider?

BC: Clinical organizations that are providing services abroad are going to have to understand how to process the local currency. You'd think that everyone should know how to do that, but when you look back at when the first businesses went global, this was the first issue they had to contend with and it was a real obstacle to getting business going.

The other big area of concern is cultural issue. We need to be thinking about when a patient goes abroad, they need to be educated on what to expect. They need to know if they'll have to stand in a line. The care is going to be different. They'll need to know that and they'll need to know how to interact with the people in a different culture.

For example, I was going to Tokyo for business and had scheduled a dinner with a group of business people. Before going, I had to learn how to interact with this group of people in this particular setting. There was the question of when to sit, who to talk to, when to get up, and so forth. And that's just for dinner. Imagine the education that will be needed to undergo a major operation!

MTT: What new types of related business or services might you expect to see evolve as the industry grows?

JV: In terms of new businesses or services, I think we can expect to see growth in the areas of international facility planning and construction. We're currently handling requests for proposals to assist companies looking to go global. Some are already to the phase of looking at architecture needs. Some are still in the strategy phase. We're helping them look at whether or not going global is an appropriate response to a competitive threat or if it's in line with their larger corporate goals. I also think we're going to see an increase need for more staff resource planning and retention.

In the past, US providers have relied heavily upon individuals trained in other countries. You're likely to see more of those clinicians choosing to stay at home and graduates of US medical schools may opt to practice abroad. This could have a very negative and serious impact on the labor supply of critical clinicians.

BC: In terms of growth opportunities, I see telemedicine as a big one. You're going to see more consultations from afar taking place as organizations try and connect with each other. I think we can also expect to see health plans offering telemedicine as part of their new products.

Additionally, there's a significant new sales channel arm being created. As mentioned before, we're seeing more and more people promoting services here in the US. They're reaching out to both employers and health plans. I think we can also expect to start seeing provider organizations begin offering concierge services for patients. By handling their travel accommodations, their transportation in the area they've traveled to, etc., they make it both easier for the client and they ensure that everything is appropriate to the type of care needed or received by the patient.

MTT: What are your biggest concerns or cautions about the industry?

JV: The whole issue of privacy and security of patient data is of major concern across the board in the US. When you take it across borders, you then have to ask who has access to my personal health records? How can you guarantee it's secure? We really need to be prepared to address threats, both real and perceived, regarding patient data.

For providers and organizations setting up practice or partnerships abroad, I think it's critical that they have a crystal clear understanding of the legal requirements of the country where they are providing care. They need to understand the requirements and balance them with US requirements.

BC: I also think there's some concern on the patient safety aspect. In the US, there's a huge emphasis on the number of errors that occur in a facility, the number of infections, and so on.

When traveling abroad, the standards of care for patients are more important. We need to consider the type of travel that will occur and the patient's condition. Furthermore, are the standards of care where they're headed the same as our own? What we don't want is the incident rates in US to rise related to problems of care received abroad when the patients return.

I think we also need to begin managing patient expectations. People, especially those who have never been abroad before and now find themselves going for the first time for a medical procedure, don't know what to expect. We'll need to rely upon the people making recommendation for travel abroad to make the effort to provide that education to patients. Otherwise, the feedback on the experience could be greatly negatively impacted -- not to mention patient recovery.

However, if we think about it as an opportunity, there are a number of content providers that provide information on procedures. We could see those content providers or others creating new content that will explain specifically what's going to happen to you when you travel abroad, specific to different countries, and so forth.

JV: Credentialing, of course is a big concern. Patients will be looking for some assurances from the JCI or elsewhere, that the quality of care is as good or better than here in the US. The credentialing process will provide that assurance that the standards of care are what's expected and desired.

MTT: Thank you both for your time and insight. It's been most informative and best of luck with efforts to help your clients grow internationally.

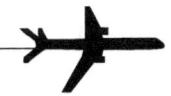

Ken Getz
Founder
Center for Information & Study of Clinical
Research Participation

February 2008

Medical Travel Today *recently had the opportunity to talk with Ken Getz, a senior research fellow at the Tufts Center for the Study of Drug Development (CSDD). In addition to his role at Tufts, Getz also runs the Center for Information & Study of Clinical Research Participation (CISCRP), a non-profit organization focused on raising public awareness and literacy for clinical research.*

> *Our conversation was interesting as it brought to light the many commonalities in the global evolution of clinical research and medical travel. We're grateful to Mr. Getz for sharing his insight and will continue to pay close attention to his industry and the lessons we can learn from it.*

Medical Travel Today (MTT): First, tell us a bit about how you got involved in clinical research.
Ken Getz (KG): My background is in management economics, psychology and the sciences. I worked in management consulting for seven years assisting mostly pharmaceutical and biotech companies in the area of research and development.

After that, I started a publishing company called CenterWatch. When the opportunity presented to sell it, I did and went on to join Tufts and start CISCRP.

The one consistent thread through all of these experiences has been clinical trials. Even while in college I participated in clinical trials. When working in consulting, I helped a company build departments and modify clinical trial practices.

MTT: Over the past few years we've all witnessed the astounding growth and acceptance of medical tourism as a viable option for consumers. How do you see or expect to see this new global approach influence the way medical trials are currently conducted?
KG: Interestingly, a lot of this has already taken place. In recent years we've seen a tremendous movement in clinical trials (FDA regulated studies) activity across the globe. Today almost half of all clinical trials are being placed in investigative sites in many parts of the world outside the US. What we're seeing now is a proliferation of companies conducting clinical testing globally. Some of the companies are absolutely huge—think big pharmaceutical companies —and others are quite small, from specialty pharmaceutical and biotechnology companies to manufacturers of herbal remedies and dietary supplements. What they're all taking advantage of is regions where there are high volumes of treatment-naïve patients and well-trained staff to run trials. India, China, Eastern Europe, and Latin America in particular are proving popular for trials. What's interesting is how the clinical trials industry and the travel medicine industry are both seeking the same types of markets—a willing consumer base and well-trained staff.

MTT: Is there potentially an opportunity for a clinical trial involving patients coming back?

KG: It's difficult to speculate or project but I suppose it's a possibility. However, you have to consider the current climate and pressure points in clinical trials. For example, as the proportion of patients getting involved in clinical trials come from regions outside the US, there's a growing pressure in the US to limit the number of trials abroad. Some people feel by going abroad we're denying US patients access to the trials.

Now what could also happen is that as American patients realize the specific clinical trial they need is not available in the US or in their part of the country, they may choose to travel to gain access. That's essentially what's happening in your industry, although getting the treatment at a given cost is the driver. It's largely the same process.

We're also seeing early signs of forces that may prompt biopharmaceutical companies to scale back the amount of clinical trials taking place overseas. Initially research sponsors moved some of their clinical trials overseas for economic reasons—they offer faster enrollment, and lower labor and operating costs.

But as the medical professionals in these regions begin to realize they can earn more then they traditionally received the economic advantages will begin to wane. Relative costs will approach parity with those of US and Western European investigators. We may see placement of clinical trials abroad begin to parody with US based trials. This is 7 to 10 years out, but that's what we need to be thinking about now.

MTT: Do you feel that medical tourism supports or hinders the work you do in any way?

KG: I see the big drivers of clinical research and medical travel being largely the same.

As consumers get savvy about treatments available only in certain markets, they begin to take more proactive and aggressive measures to gain access to these treatments.

For example a patient currently getting an asthma treatment approved two years ago could find out about a study of an experimental treatment that is potentially safer and more effective. A physician could approach them to participate and the patient could either be compensated or receive a subsidy.

You could see the same thing happening abroad. A physician could essentially recruit you and you would participate either by travel or through the Internet.

I think the industries work well in parallel. I don't see one really hurting the other. If anything, as more people get familiar with the notion of traveling abroad for medical related reasons—be it a clinical trial or a surgery—it'll make them more comfortable with the idea of traveling.

MTT: Your industry is particularly good at sharing information through forums, etc. What do you think the professionals in medical tourism could learn from that approach? What practices you think they should consider to increase consumer confidence and understanding?

KG: Well to be honest, neither the pharmaceutical or biotech industries have done a particularly good job of engaging the public. Public education simply hasn't existed and without that, public trust has deeply eroded.

I think what the medical travel industry can learn from the clinical trials industry. First and foremost, it is essential—especially with the widespread use of the Web—to put in a concerted effort to engage and educate the public. Public outreach and education cannot be overly promotional. It must be credible, and respectful. You really can't sugar coat the realities in the honest pursuit of trust.

Unfortunately, this is not the approach that the pharmaceutical industry took and, as we've discovered, it takes a lot more effort to reverse the erosion of public trust than it does to build it honestly up front.

One of the other things that pharmaceutical companies did wrong is that its conferences and communications have been very insular. The industry engaged research professionals but to a far lesser extent medical professionals. This hasn't helped to increase either acceptance or awareness.

If I were in your position, I'd seek to engage stakeholders. I'd host speakers' bureaus and lectures at medical schools and start talking to physicians. Plus, I'm a big fan of grassroots outreach efforts. If you look at the ciscrp.org Website, you'll see the types of public media programs we do. And we do these because we've found they work.

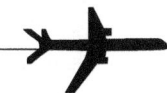

Robert M. Kolodner, M.D.
National Coordinator for HIT
Department of Health and Human Services

March 2008

Laura Carabello, Publisher of Medical Travel Today *recently had the privilege to speak with Robert M. Kolodner M.D., National Coordinator for Health Information Technology (HIT) with the Department of Health and Human Services.*

    Since joining the Department in 2006, Dr. Kolodner has made steady progress in advancing the President's Health IT initiative. Prior to joining HHS, Dr. Kolodner served as the Chief Health Informatics Officer at the Veterans Health Administration in the Department of Veterans Affairs (VA). He was involved in the development and oversight of VistA—the VA's electronic health records system—and My HealthVet—the VA's Personal Health Records for veterans.

    Medical Travel Today *spoke to Dr. Kolodner regarding his thoughts on the growth of medical travel and how players in the health information technology industry, both here in the U.S. and abroad, will need to begin to address the critical issue of medical records sharing and the impact upon patient safety.*

Medical Travel Today (MTT): What kind of, if any, international records sharing systems currently exist?
Robert Kolodner (RK): At the current time, there is none in widespread use. The problem is in the lack of standards in any one country. There are really three issues impacting internal record sharing: policies, understanding and trust.

    You've got the policies that exist in each country. Often, you've got a lack of understanding of the complexity and scope of records management. And then there's the question of trust. You need to be certain that the information is going to the right entities.

MTT: What nations outside the United States, if any, do you feel are doing the best job in terms of creating reliable systems for sharing and transferring records?
RK: In my opinion, this progress is limited to a few countries including the Netherlands, Denmark, New Zealand and the United Kingdom – and there may be others. Since adoption of electronic health records (EHR) in the United States is still at a low level, with current estimates holding that only 14 percent of providers currently have an EHR, it may be premature to advance discussions of interoperability with even those nations that are generating traction.

MTT: What obstacles currently stand in the way of creating a secure and seamless means for sharing records both domestically and across borders?
RK: Foreign countries certainly face more challenges because of the language issues. In some European countries, stakeholders have to contend with 27 or more language variations, making interoperability a significant challenge.

Some of the information translates easily. For example, with drugs, ingredients are comparable throughout the world and readily understood. Also, there are data elements and identifiers in the EHR that are fairly straightforward and not complicated by translation.

The challenge comes with progress notes. While there are incremental advances and some physicians overseas can provide care and record information in English, there's simply no reliable translator to handle this type of information. It becomes quite difficult to address the complexities and in the short term, these challenges persist.

MTT: What kind of consideration are you giving to international records sharing as you develop the Nationwide Health Information Network?
RK: We are wrestling with standards ourselves. We are not unique—others are having challenges to automate their systems. Before we can delve into international record sharing, we have to better develop what we're doing domestically.

MTT: One aspect of medical tourism that seems to be of greatest concern to doctors in the US is the after-care that returning patients may require. What are your thoughts on applying a CCR approach to this patient group?
RK: The solution should be a continuity of care (CCR) standard set by American Society for Testing and Materials (ASTM). This would be a great first step.

We need to harmonize a way of moving as much information as CCR offers but doesn't inherently make available. Groups are beginning to collaborate to bring together the best of CCR and other standards, with movement toward the common criteria document (CCD). This is where the standard is moving—incorporating the data of the CCR but enhancing it with versioning and combining it with recommendations from HL7 Groups. If an entity can transport information in a CCD format, then interim solutions such as a USB port or CD will be possible long before interoperability is achieved.

Another opportunity is for sharing-entities to introduce a portal to their systems so information can be shared. The challenge with this approach is that it may not meet the physician needs, since they can't log on to different sites.

Another solution for today's volume of patients traveling outside the country for medical care is to download their own data, print it out and carry along to the destination. This is a short-term solution and while it's not ideal, it will promote continuity of care.

We're also seeing "in-patient IT vendors" now playing in an international marketplace. They are building features into their products that may become available to promote record sharing.

We've got the beginnings of a solution in place but there are steps to go before we get there. What we need are patient-centered solutions as the industry undergoes a great deal of change and all stakeholders are focused upon patient outcomes.

MTT: Do you feel that the Department's Certification Commission might be used as a model for developing a unified set of international standards related to care provided through medical tourism?
RK: Discussion and exploration is underway with the European Union to determine areas for collaboration. But I want to stress that it's really the model of certification that we're looking at, not the certification itself.

MTT: Do you have any forecasts for the industry?

RK: Some observers think that personal health records—PHRs—may be a driving force for consumers to get their electronic health records underway. It is an interesting time for this aspect of data collection.

Everyone recognizes that the healthcare sector is dependent upon implementing sound healthcare information technology as a necessity for better care and improved outcomes. But HIT and EHRs unto themselves will not get us there.

We need to encourage every individual to understand that the quality of healthcare they receive—especially when there are multiple providers involved—is largely dependent upon physician use of EHRs to aid in the delivery and exchange of information. It is in everybody's interest to see widespread adoption of EHRs, particularly providers who want to take care of people and streamline practice workflow.

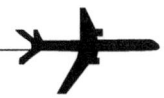

Karen Timmons
President & Chief Executive Officer
Joint Commission International

March 2008

Publisher Laura Carabello recently had the opportunity to speak with Karen Timmons, president and CEO of Joint Commission International. JCI is part of The Joint Commission, the leading accreditation organization for US hospitals. International hospitals seek accreditation to demonstrate quality, and JCI accreditation is considered a seal of approval by medical travelers from the US and patients and caregivers around the globe.

JCI has also been designated a Collaborating Centre for Patient Safety Solutions by the World Health Organization and is developing an international collaborative network to improve patient safety. Ms. Timmons is a past board member and Treasurer for the International Society for Quality in Healthcare (ISQua). What follows is part one of a two-part series featuring highlights of their conversation.

Medical Travel Today (MTT): During the recent Consumer Health World meeting in Washington, DC, a representative from one of the foreign hospitals said that JCI accreditation is another example of US imperialism. How would you respond?
Karen Timmons (KT): I don't agree with that statement. We actually like to think of ourselves as an international company, headquartered in the United States.

MTT: With the growth of medical tourism, has the JCI mission changed in any way?
KT: No, our mission has been and continues to be focused on improvement and helping organizations improve the quality and safety of the care they provide to the public. We were established in the early 1990s and started doing international work. Around 1994, our footprint expanded because many ministries of health and other key stakeholder groups that had been going to our parent company, The Joint Commission, needed assistance in developing their own national accrediting bodies or national standards to assess the quality of care within their countries or regions.

In 1999, the Joint Commission hosted 30 study tours for different countries. Literally, 30 weeks out of 52 were spent on international projects and the interest was intense. It was determined that it would be most appropriate to place those activities in the not-for-profit affiliate, then known as Quality Healthcare Resources (QHR). At that time, QHR provided technical assistance and education primarily to key stakeholders and ministries of health, helping them to establish their own national accrediting bodies or standards.

A keen interest in quality and safety evolved over the next four years, and the question of providing accreditation was presented to the Joint Commission or, more specifically, Joint Commission International (JCI). At that time, it was determined that the use of domestic standards internationally would be inappropriate, and if there was going to be the attestation of international accreditation, it should be founded upon an international set of standards that would be applicable to various countries, with their unique healthcare and delivery systems. It would need to be more sensitive to various cultural differences.

We called together a panel of about 18 different experts from around the globe, ensuring international representation from the five major regions of the world, and developed the first set of standards. Certainly, this group of experts used the framework that had been established in the domestic standards, but they really delineated any references to the national or federal agencies or things that would not be applicable internationally. There is a lot of jargon, as you can imagine, in the United States, but things such as an organized medical staff would not be applicable, as not every country has an organized medical staff.

The area such as patient consent, for example, is not always uniform. Here in the United States the individual patient would sign a consent form; that's not always the case in other countries. Different countries might have different cultures where the family might be the more appropriate body to sign consent. We developed our standards with those sensitivities in mind and, of course, the mission to help improve quality and safety has always been there.

As I said in the beginning, we view ourselves as an international company. I say that because we're not interested in just exporting the American model. We have international representation on our Board. In fact, it's a requirement in our by-laws that three board members be international members. Our standards committee is composed entirely of international experts. We also have regional advisory councils, specifically Europe, Asia-Pacific, and the Middle East. We really try to insure that we're listening to the needs, that we understand the differences of different healthcare systems, and that we learn from them.

MTT: You actually answered my second question: are the standards different for accrediting domestic versus international hospitals? Obviously they are.
KT: I would say that the standards are comparable to the Joint Commission's domestic accreditation standards. However, after we cross-referenced the standards, we recognized that they are clearly different and have been adapted for the international community. They are designed to be applicable to various cultures and healthcare delivery systems.

MTT: Do you believe the cost of accreditation is hampering foreign hospitals from achieving JCI accreditation? Is there any flexibility in pricing?
KT: Certainly, we do not believe that the cost of accreditation is hampering any major acceleration in the number of organizations seeking accreditation. I think part of that obviously has to do with the environment that you mentioned when we first started speaking. The average cost of accreditation is about $30,000, but that covers a three-year period. Obviously, that breaks down to $10,000 per year.

MTT: I dislike the word cheap—but that's cheap.
KT: Yes. And in many organizations, as you know, it really is a commitment to quality. But you have to pay for quality. To simplify it, you pay extra for cars that have the air bags on the side so…you pay for this, too.

MTT: So if you had one additional patient a year because of the accreditation, it would pay for itself. Do you agree?

KT: Well, I quoted you the average cost. But you also asked about flexibility. The fees are really based on a number of factors, including the complexity of the services offered by an organization, the number of beds and things of that nature.

MTT: How many hospitals are currently accredited? Pending?

KT: There are about 150 hospitals that are accredited right now. We have another 105 surveys this year, of which about 47 will be triennial (or re-accreditation) surveys. I would say that by the end of the year, we probably will have a little over 200 accredited.

MTT: I think there is confusion in the marketplace about the various accrediting bodies.

KT: I agree. For example, the International Society for Quality in Healthcare (ISQua) is always cited. Actually, hospitals are not ISQua-accredited. ISQua accredits accrediting bodies, and JCI is ISQua-accredited. In fact, we are a founding member of ISQua. I serve on the Board and I also serve on the Alpha Council, so we are very strong supporters of ISQua.

MTT: It's interesting, because when you ask these hospitals if they are JCI accredited, they say 'Oh no, we're not, but we meet the ISQua standards. They use that answer to convince Americans that it is some kind of accrediting body. Can you explain how ISQua operates?

KT: Sure, but first I want to make the point that I think patients and consumers should be looking for accreditation by entities that have been accredited by ISQua. You will not find a healthcare organization accredited by ISQua, only accrediting bodies.

ISQua develops the standards and principles that should guide an accrediting body on how to conduct itself. So it really is 'walking the talk' for accrediting bodies like ourselves. It requires us to put ourselves under the same scrutiny, to have the same quality improvement philosophy, and be sure that we're listening to key stakeholder groups -- just as we advise healthcare organizations to make sure that they're listening to their key customers, patients and staff.

MTT: Besides yourself, what other accreditation bodies are accredited by ISQua?

KT: There's the Australia Council, Canadian Council, the French national accrediting body called HAUTE Authority.

MTT: Let's take a moment to look at this from the consumer perspective. If the Australian Council accredits a hospital, for example, how should the American public feel about that? Should they accept that? Or should they be looking for JCI?

KT: They should be looking for Joint Commission International Accreditation because we are the premiere accrediting body and we have the highest level of standards worldwide. We are also the only accrediting body that has developed international standards. The other entities that are providing services internationally are using their own national standards.

MTT: So, Australia and Canada would be using only their national standards.

KT: Correct. We also have compared our standards to the Joint Commission's standards. We use the leading-edge survey methodology such as the tracer methodology.

MTT: What is the tracer methodology?

KT: We trace the path of a patient's journey through a hospital to ensure compliance with the standards. When doing our site visit, we would, based upon the volume of services within that organization, actually ask to see a patient's record. We'd be looking to see that the organization has filled out on their application the type of services that are provided. Suppose someone came in having a heart attack and ended up in post-surgical care: We might trace that patient back to the emergency room and as they went through the various services or procedures that they've received, we would insure compliance with our standards. We would be talking to the staff that had been taking care of that patient—how did they get consent? We would be asking whether or not they identified the patient. We trace the journey of the patient through the care they received throughout the hospital; hence, it's called tracer methodology. So it's an actual patient. Some accrediting bodies spend a lot of time looking at document reviews—they're just looking at documents of meetings and looking to see whether or not there's paper. We actually look at the care provided and what actually happens to patients. It's very care-centered, very patient-centered.

MTT: Have you ever turned a hospital down? And if so, what percentage of applicants would you say don't meet standards?

KT: Yes, we have. The number is roughly one percent. But for many organizations—especially for those that are in growth mode and first-time organizations seeking accreditation—if there is one area where they are not in compliance, we very well might ask a surveyor to go back in three months and re-evaluate them. Before we provide accreditation or give them the award of accreditation, they would have to improve their compliance.

Editors Note: *In our last issue we featured Part One of a conversation between our publisher, Laura Carabello, and Karen Timmons, president and CEO of Joint Commission International. What follows is part two of a two-part series featuring highlights of their conversation.*

MTT: There are a number of small groups currently attempting to set up some credentialing standards specifically for medical tourism. How does what you do complement these initiatives? Do you feel organizations should even consider or pursue these new standards?

KT: I believe it's very important and it's good that an organization seek external validation of the quality of its services—whether that is through accreditation, certification, ISO, etc. It's a first step and I certainly think that patients and consumers should be encouraged to seek evidence of an organization's willingness to comply with standards. I commend this and I believe that it's very important that patients look for these validations of care standards.

MTT: There are Web-based credentialing services emerging right now in the United States. Are you aware of anything that is going on internationally at that level?

KT: Not for credentialing. Our standards require that an organization have primary verification of the qualifications of its medical staff. Its physicians and other health-care clinicians have to have primary evidence that they have the credentials they indicated. They also have to be reviewed as far as the record of the quality of care that they have provided to ensure that they are qualified to provide the types of services that they've indicated they can. We would ask an organization providing the information as to whether the physician is qualified to provide a specific type of service, such as bypass surgery. Basically, it's the privileging services that you are allowing as opposed to credentialing.

MTT: If you had to look into a crystal ball, what would you say is the future of medical tourism?

KT: I think the world is very small — and this shrinking, if you will, is going to increase. I think we'll see a day, and it may very well surprise us, that people will get onto a plane and travel around the world for their specific services. It will be very much accepted, and hospitals will become procedure-driven and very expert at certain procedures. They will be specialized to provide those procedures at a high volume with high quality, and as cost effectively as possible.

MTT: What do you think the opportunities are for US-based hospitals to partner with foreign hospitals?

KT: I think hospitals around the world can share best practices. I think as the health-care industry becomes more global, there will be standardization of healthcare practices. People will want to access care from what is known as the "best" provider. Around the world, there is evidence that providers share a common goal to improve quality and safety. The sharing of these tenets on a global level is certainly helping to promote improvement.

MTT: Do you think American community hospitals or smaller hospitals should feel threatened by this whole medical tourism phenomenon?

KT: I think they should embrace it. I think it's an opportunity for uninsured and underinsured American patients who might not have access to care to get care. And I also think there's an opportunity for smaller hospitals to attract patients from abroad who come to the United States for care. For example, many Europeans come to New York, Boston and the East Coast for their care because of the favorable exchange rate.

MTT: Do you think the foreign hospitals will be able to continue to deliver the care at a lower cost?

KT: I think some of the foreign hospitals will be able to do this, especially those that are really positioning themselves as a heart hospital or are known for their care for knee procedures or hip procedures, and have really focused on how to deliver high quality care in a very efficient manner. They have worked very hard to achieve that.

MTT: Do you think that there will be any movement at all for malpractice insurance or any litigation in this arena for patients who have bad outcomes in foreign hospitals?

KT: Certainly, every country has different legal redress and there has been discussion at various conferences on whether or not there will be some sort of universal redress or common legal redress. I would assume third party payers and insurers would eventually offer some sort of protection even in the United States. If a health insurance plan is sending a patient abroad, they will have to cover some of that. It would be different for an individual person who is deciding to travel on his or her own as to what types of legal redress they might have.

MTT: What should employers and health plans in the United States look for in a foreign care provider? Is the JCI seal of approval their go ahead to use that hospital? Should they be visiting them personally?
KT: I certainly think they can seek JCI accreditation, but they should be looking for some evidence of compliance with quality standards or indicators. And the patient should also be looking for evidence of quality.

MTT: Where would a consumer find this information?
KT: Consumers need to do searches on the Web and also speak to their primary care physician. Many doctors have colleagues living and practicing abroad. I think it is very important that there be continuity of care, so they should be seeking someone who might be able to provide not only the pre-care, but also post-care, and ensure that the portability of the medical record is there.

MTT: If you had to point to one or two countries as model destinations, where would you direct attention?
KT: I certainly think that there are several countries. India, as well as Thailand, Malaysia, and Singapore have certainly positioned themselves very intentionally as sites for medical tourism.

MTT: What about places like Mexico and Guatemala that are a little closer to home? How do they stack up?
KT: Certainly, each of these countries has a certain area that positions them as a strong choice. But again, I think it's important for the consumer to look into what the organization is doing to demonstrate its commitment to quality and safety.

MTT: If you had to give a word of advice to Americans, whether it's a health plan, an employer, or the consumer-patient himself or herself, what would it be?
KT: Research, research, research. Communicate with your primary care physician and understand what you are getting into.

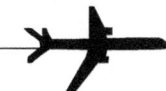

Jackie Aube
Vice President of Product Management
CIGNA HealthCare

May 2008

Medical Travel Today **(MTT): How would you define medical tourism, as the market you deal with here in the U.S. perceives it?**
Jackie Aube (JA): In my conversation with others, it's clear that the perception of medical tourism is predominantly focused on U.S.-based citizens going abroad for the purpose of medical care. Again, that's the most common definition used by individuals dealt with in the U.S.

MTT: Understanding that that's how we'll be viewing the term in the context of particular interview, can you share with me how you like the term medical tourism? Do you think it's descriptive or would you like to see something else -- is it the globalization of health care?
JA: Yes, I think a better term - and one we've actually started using internally - is global health care consumerism. I think that is a better term for how we view it here at Cigna.

MTT: Even in the context of focusing on the needs of American citizens to travel outside the country?
JA: Yes.

MTT: Do you currently have contracts with foreign hospitals to take care of your expatriates, citizens, or workers/employees that are living in other countries?
JA: Yes, we do through our Cigna international division. It's important to understand the distinction between our international division and our health care division. Through our international division we offer our employer customers the opportunity to buy expatriate coverage.

So for global companies that send their employees to other countries for business for extended periods of time, the employees will have health care coverage through our international division. We also offer products specifically designed for shorter-term assignments to allow clients to customize based on their unique needs.

MTT: So your international network is made of up the providers who offer care for employers sending employees all over the world?
JA: Yes.

MTT: Can you tell us what your U.S.-based members are looking for in terms of a care provider?

JA: Many of our customers are self-insured, which means they fund all of their claims and they have a lot of say in plan design, including specific benefits covered by the plan. I would say that employers who are considering the addition of medical tourism to their U.S.-based policies tend to be the thought leaders in the American employer-based market. They tend to be the early adopters of new trends, and we're already getting some questions regarding medical tourism and what it means for them.

We are working to develop solutions that will meet the broad range of global healthcare needs. And at this point, there is some interest in international centers of excellence. If a client is considering sending one of their employees abroad for the purpose of medical care, they are going to want to partner with a company that has experience internationally. That same company must also have the ability to consult with them about what they should be looking for in terms of facilities, safety, and quality standards—and all the other logistics you would need to think about if you were going to send an employee abroad for medical care.

MTT: If you could quantify, how many inquires would you say you've received?
JA: We've had probably 20 or so inquiries from employers and approximately 40 inquiries if you include consultants and the media. But that's just inquires— most of the employers that we have spoken to are interested in finding out more about medical tourism but haven't made the decision to add medical tourism benefits to their plan.

MTT: If you had to qualify to what extent Cigna is embracing this concept, would you say it's a low, medium, or high level? And what would be your role in making decisions related to pursuing it?
JA: My role as product lead is to monitor the trends very closely and to chart a course for Cigna that would ensure that we have solutions to meet the demand. I would say that in terms of pace, we are really letting the market drive that pace. We have received a fair amount of inquiries, but I think employers are appropriately cautious. It's very new, so we are certainly willing to work with employers that are interested in pursuing the concept further.

MTT: I want to ask you this personally because people ask me this because of the newsletter: Would you personally consider going out the country for medical care?
JA: I think if I had not been working on this particular initiative my answer would have absolutely been "No." But through the research I've been doing on behalf of Cigna, I'm now more aware of the existence of high-quality facilities outside of the US and the extent of the training of the physicians that practice in these facilities. When you consider this in addition to JCI's involvement and the pace at which several foreign hospitals are now seeking independent quality accreditations, I'd have to say that now I'm warm to the idea. Very warm.

MTT: Would you say that JCI accreditation is a must for Cigna?
JA: I wouldn't necessarily say so. I think that it always helps to have additional independent reviews, but we are still assessing what the appropriate quality indicators should be. That is probably one area where we feel there is more to do in terms of research.

MTT: I am sure you are familiar with all the other accreditation programs all over the world that seem to want to mirror JCI.
JA: Yes, I am familiar with some of them.

MTT: Given those, what countries would you say would be most appealing to Americans?
JA: We haven't completed any independent research regarding countries that would rank as most appealing to Americans, but based on employer queries, their interest tends to be focused on where the highest quality facilities are located and what a member would perceive to be high quality.

MTT: Would member perception include a language or culture?
JA: Yes. The ability to speak English is a good example. Patient perceptions begin from the point where they land at the airport until they arrive at the facility where they are going to have the procedure done.

MTT: We talked about quality as being an important factor. But obviously, cost comes into this, too. What are your thoughts on cost as a factor as it relates to quality?
JA: Cost is important. The prospect of getting on a plane and going somewhere for a medical procedure has to include some incentive. I think quality is the biggest bar to overcome because improved health is the goal of any medical procedure. People need to be assured they are going to receive high quality care first, and then the next largest factor is going to be cost – "Is it worth it for me?" Safety is also a factor. Employers need to consider any additional liabilities that they might be taking on. So, while there are several factors to consider, clinical quality and safety standards are at the top, followed by cost, and then all other implications.

MTT: Do you think there will be issues with insurance and essentially giving up your right to file a lawsuit if you had a bad outcome? Also, how does Cigna handle this matter?
JA: I do think that it's very important that if an employer intends to offer this as part of its benefit program then it needs to be made very clear to any employee who takes advantage of medical travel that the malpractice laws differ significantly between countries. U.S. medical tourists should understand that restitution for any sort of malpractice is not really matched globally.

MTT: What are the implications for Cigna? Let's say I was a Cigna member and had a bad outcome in Turkey and hold Cigna responsible for that bad outcome. Do you see that as an issue or as something this industry should tackle?
JA: I certainly think it's something that needs to be considered. I am a big fan of member education. Full disclosure of all of the benefits and risks is important, as it would be with any medical decision, and this is something Cigna would always support.

MTT: Do you currently have or plan to institute any educational sessions or focus groups for your employers or stakeholders that want to get into this?
JA: We have considered bringing interested employer groups together. In fact, it's something we are discussing right now. At this point, we are currently meeting with

employers one-on-one to determine their individual objectives, what they want to achieve, and their timelines. We intend to discern if they are just in the consideration phase or if they are ready to take action.

MTT: Are you familiar with the term value-based health design? If so, how do you see it fitting into that scenario?
JA: Yes, I'm familiar with it but I don't see much of a fit. My interpretation of value-based design is really to identify conditions where certain things like cost might prevent members from seeking the care that ultimately will lead to better health. Those types of conditions I categorize as value-based health care are more chronic conditions where ongoing compliance with maintenance medications, for example, is important to an individual's health, as opposed to the types of procedures that would be most conducive to medical tourism.

Medical tourism is most appropriate for types of procedures that don't need a lot of pre- or post-operative care, but may be high cost. Surgeries such as hip and knee replacement and some cardiac procedures—such as bypass surgery—fit this description. Value-based health designs focus on designing benefit plans intended to encourage behaviors that mitigate heath problems. For example, reducing or waiving pharmacy co-pays for drugs to lower cholesterol levels.

MTT: How about bariatrics? Are you looking at that?
JA: Bariatric or weight-loss surgery is something that really should be heavily managed both pre- and post-operative. It's really a mind-body thing. If you have bariatric surgery but have not gone through the right course of pre- and post-op treatment – including counseling for lifestyle changes and associated habits – it is not likely to be as successful, and might even be considered high-risk.

MTT: How would Cigna go about looking at after care?
JA: It is an important consideration that requires deliberate planning. This is under discussion as well.

MTT: Do you envision Cigna having a special network in place for it?
JA: We really haven't gotten that far.

MTT: That's fair. This industry is still growing up. How do you see partnerships between U.S.-based hospitals and foreign hospitals and how would that work to the benefit of a plan like Cigna? For example a Johns Hopkins might have a marketing partnership with a hospital in Singapore.
JA: I think that's a really interesting question because it is obvious that large notable facilities in the U.S. are starting to think globally, and a number of them are already creating sister partnerships internationally or have franchises internationally.

MTT: And if Cigna has contracts with those hospitals, it might be a natural extension?
JA: Yes -- it could be a natural extension if all the formal credentialing requirements were met.

MTT: If you were a gambler, what odds would you give medical tourism for acceptance in the U.S.?

JA: I view this as a trend that is going to continue to gain momentum. What I wouldn't bet on is the pace at which it will happen. I think that the momentum is going to be continually pushed by the uninsured and the underinsured because the motivation exists within this population. That same motivation just doesn't exist today in the employer-based market, so I believe the pace in that segment of the U.S. population will be slower.

MTT: Do you have any employers that have indicated they would like to get started July 1st?
JA: None that are that committed or are at that point of committing to a definite date. But we do have several customers that are actively talking about the concept.

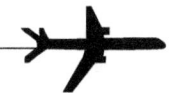

Steven Tucker
President & Medical Director
The International Medical Travel Association

At the recent Consumer Health World conference in Las Vegas, The International Medical Travel Association (IMTA) debuted its American presence. Medical Travel Today recently had the opportunity to talk with the IMTA's president and medical director, Dr Steven Tucker, MD (USA), FACP (USA) about this development, their plans for growth within the U.S. and other countries, as well as his perspective on the industry as a whole.

Medical Travel Today (MTT): Very exciting news about your U.S. presence. Can you tell us a bit about what drove the decision to establish that presence and what your intents for growth in the U.S. might be?
Steve Tucker (ST): As I see it, there are currently three types of medical travel taking place: regional medical travel, travel to centers of excellence, and most recently medical travel from North America to other destinations such as Asia and South America. All these patients are seeking high quality care at a better price point.

Recall that medical travel is not a new concept. For years, people have been traveling from Europe, Asia, the United Kingdom, and so on to other destinations for medical and dental care abroad. But now, there's an increased awareness of medical travel in the U.S. for obvious reasons.

The International Medical Travel Association (IMTA) is an international body, and we need a strong presence in all countries. Because of the growing interest in the U.S., it seemed to us to be the next logical beachhead for expanding our outreach. Plus, as part of our mission, we need to find as many common touch points as possible with medical travel players across the world. There are so many emerging players in the U.S. that it also made it a great choice.

As an aside, and this is a personal opinion, global medical travel, unlike the U.S. medical system, presents an opportunity to make the healthcare industry work like it should: a system where physicians and providers can determine their value in an open and transparent environment; an environment where patients have opportunities for choice in the medical services they receive; and a reduction, and in some cases a complete elimination, of the number of third-party payors involved.

When you have that, you have a very real value proposition. And when it's done well, everyone is satisfied with the quality services provided and received.

MTT: Do you have any plans for establishing a presence in other countries?
ST: Not at the moment. We have not established a timeline for creating a presence in another continent or country. Part of our reason for choosing the United States was that so many of our constituents are either interested in North America or have been approached by potential North American partners.

Ultimately, we need to spend more time in Europe and South America. And we'll get there. But growth for growth's sake really isn't a part of our mission. We're a young organization and strictly run through volunteerism. We need to make sure we're a sustainable association so we can continue down the path of our 'patient first' approach and keep moving our constituents in that direction. Plus, we're really looking to connect people who need each other. The globalization of health-care services is happening, and we need a body around it to make sure it stays at the highest level. That's what we're trying to do. That's our focus.

MTT: How large is the IMTA at this time and what regions or countries do the members represent?
ST: Right now we're at around 35 members, although we expect that number to double in next six months. Our goal is to reach 100 members by 2009. As for where they're from, if you asked me six weeks ago I would have told you most were from Southeast Asia. But now we represent Southeast Asia, some European countries, the U.S., and South and Central America. Our biggest increase has definitely come from the U.S. and Mexico.

MTT: What are you doing or planning to do to attract members and growth in South and Central America as well as Europe?
ST: Central and South America is on our radar for a lot of reasons. First, there is something like 50 million Spanish-speaking Americans. Second, Mexico and South America have quality services, and they fully understand travel and needs of medical travelers. Add to that the fact they are contiguous to the U.S., and they are doing what's needed to drive medical travel. Of course this is all driven by the frustrations Americans have with access to the U.S. health-care system. Americans spend more than anyone else in the world on health care and yet the dissatisfaction rate is incredibly high.

Other countries are simply doing it better on many levels. Around the world, they are providing just honest-to-goodness care—doctors who call their patients, attentive nurses, and great care. When an American patient has that kind of interaction, they are shocked. It's simply a level of care they are not used to. Honestly, they're shocked.

As for our approach to these markets, we're a little more laissez faire about membership. Right now we are interested in networking key players and new players. We don't have an aggressive media program, and we're not "out there" marketing. But we're also not being a wallflower either. We're an association that's interested in people and businesses who are interested in what we are doing. We're not looking to simply drive membership numbers. We're interested in the quality of our members and the quality of services and value we bring to them as members.

We've got some serious regional players—Parkway, Bumrungrad, Wocroft—and I expect we'll see more like that coming on board soon.

MTT: Coming off of the Vegas conference and the IMTA's U.S. debut, what are your thoughts on the future of the industry both short- and long-term?
ST: The industry of "medical tourism" itself is not going away. Call it what you will – globalization, medical travel, or outsourcing -- the industry is health-care delivery, plain and simple. All that's changing is that people are willing to travel greater distances or can now travel with greater ease than in the past to access the best medical care.

In the short-term, there will most certainly be an increase in the number of medical travelers. We're going to see more and more. The recent McKinsey report indicated the numbers are small for intensive and complex inpatient surgeries, but they defined the population of their research very specifically and only looked at that population. They didn't consider, for example, the 400,000 people traveling to Singapore from Indonesia, for routine care and mid-level procedures. The McKinsey definition of medical traveler was very tight, very specific. But still you cannot deny that these other cases constitute the bulk of medical travel.

But even with their small number, they concluded that the potential is huge. Now use a larger, and what I think is a more accurate, denominator in that equation and it's not just huge; it's a staggering number of medical travelers.

In what I'll call the mid-short term, say five to ten years, I do think you'll see a decrease in the industry. Around the world, we should be able to create better health-care services in those locations from which people are currently departing.

Take Vietnam. Right now a majority of their health care is exported. But give it another five years and they'll be able to provide a higher quality of care. Many of those patients won't go abroad for care. They'll have as good or better care options close to home.

Over in the U.S., I suspect we'll see a reduction in the cost of care. After the system breaks, and it will, we'll see a shift toward transparency on the finance side of health care. That transparency will lead to change. We'll see big decreases in the cost of care. It could be as much as fifty percent depending upon procedures, especially for electives. I'm a big believer that people value products and services most when they pay directly for them. Conversely, people don't appreciate a service or product when it has no perceived cost to them. American patients clearly need to re-evaluate their sense of quality care. I believe that's definitely going to happen. Patients will begin to appreciate a famous quote from Warren Buffet, and that is "Price is what you pay. Value is what you get."

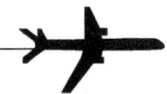

Sharon Kleefield
Faculty
Harvard Medical School

June 2008

Sharon Kleefield, former director of Healthcare Quality at Harvard Medical International and currently on the faculty of Harvard Medical School, first became interested in medical travel two years ago when a former colleague asked her to do some investigation on this subject. That investigation provided important insights regarding international medical travel and patient care and the need for ensuring patient safety and quality of care around the globe. Medical Travel Today *recently had the opportunity to talk with her about that vision and her plans for making it a reality.*

Medical Travel Today (MTT): First, can you tell us a bit about the nature of the research you were doing that spurred your interest in medical travel?
Sharon Kleefield (SK): Certainly, but first let me mention that I had done a lot of work previously in countries such as India and Thailand, where much of today's medical travel is taking place. So even when I first began the research, I was already familiar with how the industry worked and who the key players were in the field.

That said, I was asked by a colleague from a major U.S. insurance company to look into the growing trend of patients traveling outside of the U.S. for care and to offer a way of assessing the quality of the care at the centers with the largest volume of patients. This was strictly exploratory, not implementation.

As I started to do the research, I didn't see a way of comparing or contrasting different hospitals or hospital systems from the patient's perspective. I was approaching it based on the value equation. That is, "Yes, I can save and probably afford a hip resurfacing procedure, but how do I know I'll get the best quality?"

I decided to contact individuals who were already involved in the industry to ask them how they were doing it or would do it. I sent inquiries and found wide variations in approach to the question.

I didn't get anything specific back, but I did get a lot of responses saying, "This is a really important question, and we really need to figure this out. Let us know if you do."

MTT: So that continues to be the question you're looking to answer?
SK: Yes, but my interest now is more than just research-based. It's also practical. I'm in the process of formalizing a group of insurers and providers who can get together and actually build consensus on a set of measures or indicators that would provide a window on care at their location.

MTT: Similar to what JCI is doing?
SK: Yes and no, in that I feel very strongly that this needs to be created by the provider institutions, rather than by an outside organization. They need to develop a set of indicators that would be specific to the provision of care across the hospital, but

also measures that would be specific to a small set of procedures that are offered to international patients. I'm looking at those that are increasing in number and are more risky for patients, such as hip replacement, hip resurfacing, knee replacement, coronary artery bypass, and valve replacement with a critical view of issues related to appropriateness and continuity of care.

Getting back to the JCI, the hospitals that reach a level of five-star or are the centers of excellence are those that have been accredited by the JCI, or other regional or local accrediting bodies. That's really the baseline. But none of those accreditations get at the specific kind of indicator measures that go deeply into a stratification of a set of patients by procedure. Their accreditations are more general in nature.

The next level, the one I'm looking to help create, is one that can produce data. What I would call evidence-based indicators related to, not just international patients but to the total number of patients getting those procedures as a whole stratified by procedures and outcomes at a given facility.

So if I needed a knee replacement, I would be able to find out that if I go to, for example, a Bumrungrad or Wockhardt, I would know that during the last year or two they've done a given number of knee replacements. And then, what does that mean? Who are the physicians performing most of the procedures? What are the credentials of the physicians? What are the patient outcomes of the procedure? What are the complication rates? What are the infection rates? – just to to suggest a few questions.

MTT: Essentially, patients will have two tiers of quality measures to look at—JCI or a local accrediting body and then the measures you'd provide. Is that correct?
SK: Right. The first level would be an accreditation level they would look for, and then we would provide information based on the institution's track record for specific procedures. Only institutions that maintain such data sets would be evaluated. It would give them a good benchmark, as well.

MTT: Do you have an idea of where this organization might be centered and who might be involved?
SK: Right now I'm trying to figure out how it would be structured and centered. It might initially be developed through an established organization or through what I would call a "consensus group." It would be made up of individuals who are involved in providing care for these patients, and are interested in performing health-services research in their hospital.

Many people are interested because it's needed. Being able to measure quality and safety in a data-driven way is needed. I've given several talks at meetings on the subject and am getting a core group of people interested. And I have been working closely with a private hospital group in India that not only carries international accreditation, but also a large enough data set to measure quality and safety for their patients undergoing these procedures. Those are the types of organization and individuals I'm looking to involve.

MTT: What's your timeframe for bringing a formalized group together?
SK: I hope to pull together a group in Singapore in February 2009, in conjunction with a conference. I'm also looking to do a workshop or hold group discussions on the subject, to start people thinking and moving towards developing skills in this area.

MTT: It would seem from all that you're doing you see the potential for a lot of continued growth in medical tourism.

SK: Well, yes, but I don't know that it's necessarily going to come from the United States. The latest McKinsey study showed that the rate of growth isn't necessarily what some anticipated. On the other hand, if you speak to Kurt Schroeder from Bumrungrad, he'll tell you he's seeing more and more patients each month. The same is true at Wockhardt in India.

So again, I don't know how long it will take this industry to grow. If we had a significant change in the healthcare policy in the U.S., it's better to keep patients here. On the other hand, there are plenty of other patients from other countries who would take advantage of care abroad because the standard of care might be lacking in their own country.

So I think there is growth potential but not necessarily from the U.S.

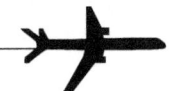

Wouter Hoeberechts
Chief Executive Officer
WorldMedAssist

September 2008

Recently, Swiss Re's Commercial Insurance announced that it had selected WorldMedAssist (www.worldmedassist.com) as the company's preferred partner to provide medical logistics to manage the medical travel options for current and future policyholders.

Medical Travel Today had the opportunity to speak with Wouter Hoeberechts, CEO of WorldMedAssist, to learn more about his company and its new relationship with Swiss Re.

Medical Travel Today (MTT): Tell me about your new partnership with Swiss Re and how it came about.

Wouter Hoeberechts (WH): Yes, we signed a contract with Swiss Re a couple of weeks ago. It's exciting because it's the first time a major U.S. insurer committed to being active in medical tourism on a national level. It is the critical step required to enable employers to reduce their medical costs by offering high quality, lower cost medical procedures outside the United States.

As one of the leaders in the medical tourism industry, we are fortunate to have been considered for a partnership by many institutions. Swiss Re sent us a request for proposal (RFP) at the end of 2007. It was a very intensive process. They truly did their due diligence on us spanning more than seven months, and at the end of the day, we were chosen as their partner.

MTT: Can you tell us about the RFP? What were they looking for? How many other companies were in the running

WH: I'm not sure exactly how many companies received the original RFP, but I do know that there were several rounds with strict requirements for each round. In terms of what they were looking for, it was a very, very in-depth and extensive review process.

There were a lot of questions around the vision of our company. What's our philosophy? Our motto? What do we think the future will look like? They were looking to make sure that we were on the same page now and in the future.

Our focus on customers is absolutely number one with us. We're committed to doing everything ethically. And that's not just marketing fluff. We were actually the first ones in the industry to publish a set of ethical guidelines (http://www.worldmedassist.com/medical_tourism_guidelines.htm).

Our service edge comes from making things easy and patient advocacy. Swiss Re asked us a lot of questions in both areas.

They were also concerned about how we select hospitals. They wanted to know that there was a true process and we weren't working with just anybody that contacted us. I think the fact that we have just five hospitals we work with speaks to the fact that we're very selective.

Our philosophy behind the small number is that we want to partner with only the highest quality providers, and we want to keep the number limited so that we truly have a partnership with them. We're not looking for someone to just have a transaction with but rather, a partner who wants to make things better for patients as much as we do.

In fact, in addition to resolving issues on an ad hoc basis, each quarter we work with our partner hospitals to look at specific instances and trends. We tell them where we'd like them to improve and note where they did well. Obviously, we know we can always improve as well so we ask for open feedback.

They're very receptive to the feedback. After all, they know we have the ears of the patients so they want to listen and make the necessary changes. That entire process was very important to Swiss Re. Also, we provided a lot of quality data from our partner hospitals. That made Swiss Re very comfortable.

There were also questions around our team. We have an excellent team. We have nurses instead of sales people doing case management, a medical doctor on staff, marketing staff, and communications people. And since earlier this year we've had staff targeting the institutional market. The person in charge of this market came to the position with 30 years of experience in the insurance field, so he can speak the language and fully understands the issues of the market.

There was also a lot of discussion about liability protection. How are we protected, the Health Insurance Portability and Accountability Act (HIPAA) requirements, and so forth.

My background is in process improvement and strategic management consulting. So our company's processes are documented, very well organized, and we have a scalable model that's ready to grow. This is true for our information technology (IT) infrastructure as well. We have proprietary software that allows us to grow quickly.

Plus, there was good chemistry. Right from the start it felt right. I think we all felt like, "Yeah, this is a good fit and we can work together." On Swiss Re's list of "must haves," we came out on top.

MTT: Are you the only provider their members can work through in order to be covered?
WH: We're the preferred provider. A client could work with another medical travel company, but we're the one Swiss Re will refer people to when asked. Similarly, if a company comes to us looking for a re-insurer, we would refer them to Swiss Re.

MTT: How have things changed for you since the announcement?
WH: Prior to the press release being issued, we received a lot of what I call tire-kicking calls. These were from all players in the institutional market: insurance companies, third party administrators (TPA), brokers, and employers. Since the press release, the volume of inquiries is up, and it's definitely more than tire kicking. Now these conversations are moving forward and moving quickly.

MTT: Are you finding more insurance companies are open to medical travel?
WH: Definitely. Last year we had a lot of interest but it was at a very basic level. Sort of a 'what is this thing called medical travel?' kind of query. Then at the start of this year, the questions became much more in-depth in nature. They're asking about rate structures and quality indicators. They are much more serious now. Interest is up and so is understanding.

MTT: Obviously insurance coverage has been an obstacle for consumers, and this new product, to some extent, removes it. I'm interested in your perspective as a facilitator about what other major obstacles still exist for the consumer interested in accessing global care.

WH: I think the biggest obstacle—the issues around liability protection—will resolve itself when the insurance companies get involved. And as we've seen, that's already happening.

Other than that, education is the biggest obstacle. It really is a nascent market that has had a tremendous amount of buzz. However, there are a still a lot of people out there who have never heard of medical tourism or have misconceptions about how it works and what risks are involved.

We need to look at raising awareness and increasing education. The fundamentals of what we do are so good that there really aren't a lot of changes needed on the execution side. We just need to make sure consumers, employers, insurance brokers, and insurance companies truly get it.

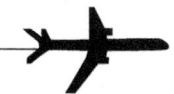

Matt Leming
Vice President & National Sales Director
Swiss Re

Medical Travel Today **(MTT): Tell us about what kinds of trends and data prompted Swiss Re to add medical travel coverage to your offerings?**
Matt Leming (ML): We really started well over a year ago. One of the issues we were primarily concerned with was how to help employer groups control cost. Claim expenditures are continuing their steep rise. One study we prepared reported a rise of inpatient hospital expenses up 170 percent during a six-year period. Obviously, there's a tremendous need to contain costs. Add to that the fact that employers are looking for employees to contribute more to the cost while others are eliminating benefit plans altogether. We see medical travel as a way to help employers help employees.

MTT: Was the decision in any way prompted by employer demand?
ML: What we continue to see is that there's a portion of the under- and uninsured marketplace that's already utilizing the medical travel option. These individuals are looking for care at affordable prices so that they can obtain procedures they need but cannot afford in the United States.

Our focus is the insured marketplace. We're interested in how we can bring this additional choice for employees to employers with self-funded plans. I can't say that we had employer demand when we started product development, but there was considerable market interest. We bring medical travel to our clients as another option to consider for their benefit plans.

MTT: Do you anticipate people utilizing the coverage for particular types of services or treatments?
ML: Today, our medical travel product is based upon covered procedures in the employer's plan document. If the procedure is not currently covered, it will not be covered under the medical travel option. It's the employee's choice of whether or not to utilize this benefit under the employer's plan. There is a possibility that employers may consider offering a medical travel option for procedures not covered under their plan document, however, this is not the primary purpose of this offering.

MTT: What can you tell us about the process of choosing a medical logistics partner? What were the capabilities or approach you were looking for?
ML: I can only discuss this at a high level due to the fact that we have signed confidentiality agreements with companies involved in the review. I can tell you that it was a rigorous process. Philosophically, our search criteria looked closely at the approach of the logistics facilitator and the business of medical travel. We also looked closely at whom they worked with and how they got their business. We needed to know what quantifiable data they used to select their overseas providers. We were also very interested to know how they could grow with us. Really, we looked at every possible aspect

of their business and how they would integrate with our business model. We did this over a six-month period and, as I said, it was rigorous.

We approached 10 U.S.-based companies with a Request For Information (RFI) initially and ultimately pared it down to just one: WorldMed Assist.

MTT: Recognizing that it has only been a few months since you've begun offering the product, can you tell us what kind of response you've received thus far?
ML: There's definitely been interest in the marketplace. But it is still nascent. Most employer groups are still trying to wrap their arms around exactly what it is. There's a lot of education that still needs to take place. On our end, we've conducted several webinars with existing clients, and we when we meet with our clients, we spend time educating them about medical travel – what it is, what it offers them as an employer, how it works for their employees. There's also the education of how a logistics facilitator helps with the process. This is completely new to many folks.

MTT: What's your understanding of how other insurers are approaching the medical travel market?
ML: I actually just sat on a panel with some folks from Assurant, CIGNA, Aetna, and others at the World Medical Tourism Congress in San Francisco. The big difference between Swiss Re and the others is that we reimburse plans at an excess level and are not a first-dollar carrier. I don't know their specific plans or schedule, but I can say that the direct carriers are still researching how they will include and integrate overseas provider networks into existing networks. They also have to look at how they'll account for quality. They have a whole list of issues to address in terms of quality of care that we rely on WorldMed Assist to accomplish. The prevailing attitude is that this is a market that's moving forward, and people are looking for ways to maximize benefits or make their dollar stretch further. The insurance organizations do recognize the market's potential.

MTT: From your perspective, what possible obstacles exist for the growth of medical travel?
ML: The one thing I see that has the greatest potential to slow the growth of medical travel is the issue of medical malpractice. What happens if something happens to me abroad? This is a question that needs to be addressed by the consumer, the employer, and the insurer. We really need to understand what rights an individual has overseas. But really, so much is dependent upon the marketplace—their acceptance and interest in the opportunity of medical travel. One really good thing, in my opinion, is the American Medical Association's issuance of guidelines for medical travel. They see it happening, and they've evaluated the opportunity and have offered constructive guidelines for both U.S. providers and consumers. Hopefully, that will impact consumer confidence.

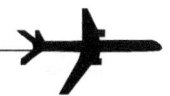

Mack Banner
Chief Executive Officer
Bumrungrad International, Bangkok

December 2008

Medical Travel Today **(MTT): How would you characterize the market for U.S. medical travelers accessing care at Bumrungrad?**

Mack Banner (MB): Bumrungrad became a pioneer in the U.S. medical travel market following the opening of our current large facility in 1997. Over the past 11 years the number of U.S. patients seen in our hospital has steadily grown. Last year, of the more than 425,000 international patients (almost 1,200 international patients per day) we served, approximately 62,000 from the United States. Of those 62,000 Americans about 50 percent actually got on a plane and came from the United States, and the other half were U.S. expatriates living in the region. We are now considered one of the anchor international hospitals by those who are in the business of medical travel due to our size, quality, and the scope of services we offer, as well as the reputation we've earned caring for international patients over the years.

Bumrungrad is a private sector hospital, with 554 licensed beds and 190 outpatient clinics seeing approximately 3,000 patients every day – 40 percent of these are non-Thais, including medical travelers, resident expatriates, and individuals from surrounding countries. About 72 percent of patients fall into the self-pay category, with the rest being covered by their employer, insurance, or government agency contracts from around the world. The current facility opened in 1997 and was the first of its kind worldwide: a large-scale operation with impressive capabilities that triggers a real WOW reaction from first time patients and visitors.

MTT: Please describe Bumrungrad's rise in the international health care marketplace.

MB: Back in 1997 during the Asian financial crisis, local demand for private health care services had dried up and forced management to look outside the immediate area for patient visits. The silver lining to the Baht's devaluation was that for those paying in U.S. currency we became half price overnight. Upper income patients from surrounding countries, including Cambodia and Bangladesh, also began utilizing the hospital in their quest for higher quality healthcare. During this time, our hospital began to emerge as one of the preferred private hospitals in Asia, a role formally held by the Mt. Elizabeth Hospital in Singapore.

After 9/11, patients from the Middle East found it increasingly difficult to get visas to travel to the United States and Europe, so they began utilizing our hospital. In 2001, we treated approximately 12,000 patients from the Middle East; this year we will provide services to more than 100,000 patients from there. Today, for many patients from the Middle East we are their general hospital and a mainstream provider of care. Of course, there is always competition, particularly as Dubai develops some impressive facilities and attracts some Middle Easterners to migrate back home. Others are also trying to woo patients, including Bangkok General Hospital. Singapore hospitals are attracting patients from Southeast Asia, Vietnam, and Cambodia while hospital companies from India are setting up hospitals Sri Lanka and Bangladesh. We are no longer alone in this international marketplace – everyone has an interest.

MTT: Has the marketplace changed significantly over the past year? Please describe.
MB: Two major changes have occurred over the past few of years. First, medical Travel intermediaries, both real and virtual, have materialized along with medical travel associations. And sometimes it seems like there are even more medical travel conferences than patients! Secondly, global care options are now becoming available, with increasing numbers of insurance companies announcing plans to provide coverage for what we have termed the "global care option" as part of their mainstream health care plans in the United States.

MTT: What are the key areas of medical excellence for Bumrungrad? Has this changed in the past year or do you expect changes?
MB: We are known for our extensive array of excellent subspecialty medicine services, with a distinctive reputation for heart, cancer, orthopedics, and other advanced specialties. Our Centers of Excellence also attract Americans and others who are considered "accidental tourists": people who did not make the trip for healthcare, but decided they needed or wanted care when they arrived – say, because they got sick or had an accident.

The serious medical travelers come for a specific procedure, driven by the cost savings. A hip replacement that would run $50,000 in the United States costs $15,000 here. While cost savings vary according to procedure, they are typically 30 to 70 percent below U.S. pricing. The differentials are higher for more complex procedures.

Clearly, the opportunity for savings is a major driver of the globalization of healthcare, with insurers and employers looking to waive deductibles and co-pays or pay for lodging to incentivize employees to take advantage of opportunities outside the United States.

MTT: Why should Americans regard Bumrungrad as a preferred option for medical care?
MB: We have more than 1,000 doctors on our staff; more than 200 of these doctors are U.S. board certified. Many of them also serve as faculty members at one of three leading medical universities here in Bangkok. Our doctors cover all major specialties and, with their clinics all located here at our hospital, it is like having a very large multi-specialty group practice: a one-stop shop for almost any condition a patient might face. When necessary, patients can usually see multiple specialists, have all their diagnostic work-ups completed, and receive their outpatient treatments and medications in one day.

In 2002, we became the first hospital in Asia to achieve accreditation from the Joint Commission International (JCI) and have been re-accredited twice. This year, the JCI survey team used their newly updated standards and the tracer methodology; these surveys are now very similar to the extensive surveys conducted by JCI's sister organization in the United States for accrediting hospitals there.

Bumrungrad now has an extensive array of international patient support services including:

1. An International Medical Coordination Office: a team of seven doctors and 20 nurses who cater to the special needs and requests of our non-Thai patients.
2. A large e-mail management team that responds to 300 to 500 e-mail inquiries daily, typically with responses within 24 hours.
3. Extensive English-speaking staff, complemented by more than 100 interpreters.
4. Airport meet-and-greet services to guide patients through immigration and arrange transport to their hotel; we have two hotels on campus and a wide variety of other hotels (at all price ranges) within easy walking distance.
5. Concierge services; Wi-Fi throughout the hospital; rentable laptop computers.
6. An extensive selection of international restaurants (including McDonald's and Starbucks) on our campus.

We update our Web site (www.bumrungrad.com) constantly to provide our international patients with extensive information about our hospital, doctors, procedures, and programs online. Last month we introduced a feature called REALCOST. This is a feature providing information on the actual costs our patients paid for 45 of our most popular procedures and examinations. These costs include all costs associated with the care, including all hospital, medication, procedure and room fees, doctor fees, and so on. We feel this program will become the world standard in providing cost information for patients. It addresses what we've seen from some hospitals that only provide partial or "lowball" estimates in order to attract patients to their facilities.

A multi-national professional management team with American, British, Australian, Malaysian, and Singaporean executives complements our core Thai team of senior executives.

MTT: What U.S. networks, health plans, or employers does Bumrungrad maintain relationships with for medical travel?
MB: We have a pioneer agreement with Blue Cross and Blue Shield of South Carolina, which was signed last year, and we now have an agreement with Companion Global Care. Overall, we have in place about ten specific agreements with eight different companies and their different subsidiaries, such as AIG, United, Cigna, and Blues plans. We have working relationships with 15+ U.S. insurance companies and third party administrators. We deal with many intermediaries – some with actual offices, some with virtual or Internet-based locations. In the United States we have no preferred medical travel partners and no appointed agent, but we do work with and are supportive of many of the groups now offering medical travel related services. While formal agreements may not be in place, we are pretty flexible and have accepted their guarantees of payment on a case-by-case basis. We receive a significant number of calls and e-mails and have more than 20 people responding to these requests. The daily volume of inquiries ranges from 300 to several thousand when a story breaks in the media.

MTT: Is JCI accreditation of importance and why?
MB: Of the many thousand international hospitals in the world, the JCI has now accredited about 197 institutions. The JCI accreditation program is now the "gold standard" for measuring the quality of hospital operations throughout the world. The JCI accreditation program is modeled after the U.S. Joint Commission on the Accreditation

of Healthcare Organizations (JCAHO); in its own way, this is as rigorous an evaluation for an international hospital (in key clinical areas) as the JCAHO is for U.S. hospitals.

MTT: Does Bumrungrad offer significantly lower costs for high quality medical care?

MB: YES! As stated earlier, our costs will generally range from 30 to 70 percent less than U.S. hospital costs, depending on the type of procedure. The cost savings generally are much more for the higher end, more complex procedures and the higher end diagnostic procedures. Our Web site features REAL costs for surgical and diagnostic procedures, reflecting actual prices paid by patients during the past year for 45 of our most popular procedures and tests. We want the cost of care to be totally transparent and expect that prospective patients will want to see what others have paid. People need transparent, unvarnished data. Our average costs are a bit less than in Singapore and a bit more than in India.

However, a sometimes-overlooked cost factor when considering care in a foreign country is the cost of the after-discharge lodging and food prior to flying home. This can normally be one to two weeks or more, depending on the complexity of the procedure. Earlier this year we went online to compare the cost of a week's lodging and food – using their best daily rate including breakfast and the cost of the lunch and dinner buffets at their coffee shops -- at the Marriott Hotel near our hospital against the Marriott Hotel in Singapore, which was located near one of our competitors. We found the cost to be about $102 USD less per day to stay here in Bangkok than in Singapore. We then did a similar comparison with a Sheraton hotel in New Delhi and were surprised to find that the hotel cost in India was about $200 USD per day higher than here in Bangkok.

MTT: Does Bumrungrad offer any options for insurance (malpractice) coverage?

MB: All of our physicians and our hospitals maintain full malpractice insurance coverage. However, it is important for international patients to know and accept that any dispute regarding care or outcomes in an international hospital will be resolved in the jurisdiction (and country) of the hospital, not the home country of the patient.

Thailand has a professionally transparent legal system and patients have access to dispute resolution procedures available through the Thai Medical Council. Penalties for malpractice can include loss of license to practice; however, American patients should know that malpractice awards in Thailand are generally much lower than those awarded in the United States.

MTT: Will Bumrungrad share its outcome data?

MB: We routinely share our outcome data with insurance companies and other corporate organizations that make inquiries.

Bumrungrad has made the following recommendations for international hospitals regarding reporting of outcomes:

- Adopt ICD-10 and CPT Coding for all discharges and procedures
- Capture experience statistics for both hospital and key doctors for high profile procedures and diagnoses
- Capture 50 percent and 90 percent of costs on acuity-adjusted discharge data

- Develop and record condition specific clinical criteria for selected procedures and diagnoses
- Capture overall patient satisfaction rates by diagnosis
- Profile international patient handling infrastructure

MTT: What is your vision for Bumrungrad regarding medical travel?

MB: We are planning to more than double our clinical capacity in the next three years while significantly enhancing the personal experience for our international and local patients.

With the potential "tipping point" of insurance-sponsored patients taking advantage of the global care option, we are preparing for the potential of significant increases in higher acuity patients being served by our hospital. We are ready – but this "tipping point" hasn't happened yet, and we're not banking on it for 2009.

The economic meltdown that is now occurring should play in favor of medical travel. It's still a question of whether American patients will do nothing, opt for somewhat elective or discretionary procedures, or simply delay care. Nobody knows the timeframe.

Today, people are worried about keeping their own jobs, and medical travel may be controversial. We estimate that it takes about a year for an insurance company to make a decision regarding developing a global patient option insurance plan offering: they first have to see the facility, then convince their boss that it is a quality destination, convince a committee, and then get their lawyers to review. This is not an overnight process.

Also, we continue to expand our representative offices into new markets. We are committed to being one of the most advanced hospitals in the world for the coming decade in regards to information technology.

Last year, Microsoft purchased our hospital's totally integrated hospital information system (HIS) from our sole-source vendor and entered into a long-term affiliation agreement to further develop this software in the coming years in collaboration with our Bumrungrad team. Our advanced capabilities will enable us to maintain state-of-the-art communication of medical data and records with both home country providers as well as electronic claims administration by international insurance companies.

MTT: What is your perspective on the associations that are now getting organized for the industry?

MB: We belong to both the Medical Travel Association (MTA) and the International Medical Travel Association (IMTA). Both these organizations play an emerging role in the further development of this whole field of medical travel and global care options. My view is that their value is similar to an industry-specific chamber of commerce: to serve as a clearing house of ideas, information, and innovations to enhance the professionalism of the sector as well as further the business objectives of its members and stakeholders.

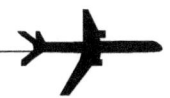

Cathy Sullivan Clark
Senior Principal
Noblis Center for Health Innovation

January 2009

Cathy Sullivan Clark is a senior principal at the Noblis Center for Health Innovation. Clark and her colleagues at Noblis have been keeping a close watch on the current and potential impact of medical travel on U.S. providers and hospitals. Medical Travel Today *recently had the opportunity to talk with her about the opportunities and challenges medical travel presents.*

Medical Travel Today (MTT): Tell us how you foresee the surge in medical travel impacting U.S. health providers.
Cathy Sullivan Clark (CSC): First, I'd like to talk about the reality of a dramatically changing competitive landscape. In the past, it was easy to define health care competition in terms of simple geography. A hospital's primary competitors were other hospitals across town or within an hour's or a few hours' drive. Today, the competition may not only be across the street, but also across the ocean, and geography is no longer the barrier to entry that it was in the past. In this respect, medical travel adds a huge level of uncertainty for U.S. hospitals. As long as competitors were in a clearly prescribed geographic area, it was relatively easy to stay on top of what those competitors were doing and how to respond appropriately. With medical travel, this simple view of competition goes out the window.

Medical travel also has the potential to create significant challenges for hospitals in managing their overall service portfolios. Medical travel is essentially creating new, non-traditional competition for those medical procedures and services that have been, at least historically, the most profitable for hospitals. These include various orthopedic and cardiac procedures, cosmetic surgeries, and weight loss surgeries among others—the very service lines on which many hospitals rely to ensure their overall financial viability. Many individual health services are not profitable but are essential to meeting community needs. The only way a hospital can afford to maintain these services is by offering other services that do generate a return. The risk to the community is that if a hospital doesn't have enough profit areas, it can't meet community needs. Medical travel is a significant threat to hospitals seeking to maintain a balanced portfolio of services—including both self-sustaining services and those that are not.

MTT: What are your thoughts on how medical travel might grow?
CSC: I believe that medical travel has the potential to grow substantially as long as there is a big price differential between services offered here at home and services offered elsewhere. As consumers take on larger and larger out-of-pocket costs for the healthcare they use, they will look more closely at the value of what they're getting. While quality concerns may have been a barrier to medical travel in the past, these concerns are disappearing. For me, medical travel is the ultimate reflection of con-

sumerism in healthcare. Based on information regarding quality and price, consumers are voting with their feet.

The current state of our economy and the economic crisis we're all facing also could facilitate greater medical travel. With less discretionary income, patients in the United States will be more interested in alternatives—medical travel included.

How fast medical travel grows will depend in part on the position that employers and payers take. If they take a more active role in encouraging patients to consider medical travel, we should expect more rapid growth. Until now, medical travel has been fueled mainly by "pull strategies:" -- approaches that attract the end user by virtue of reputation and/or the cost/quality equation. Push is about the channels of distribution that funnel patients to a particular provider. When employers start promoting medical travel, that's a push strategy. As the number of employers pushing medical travel increases, so should its popularity.

MTT: Is there a way hospitals can overcome these challenges?
CSC: I see several potential paths for U.S. hospitals facing competition from medical travel.

First, hospitals in this country must continue to innovate—to find smarter, better, and more cost-effective ways of delivering exceptional care. They must be able to compete effectively on both quality (clinical outcomes) and service (the patient experience). They need to offer the same amenities available elsewhere and pay close attention to what matters most to patients. To the extent that medical travel is setting a new standard for service, hospitals in this country will at least need to match it.

U.S. providers must also focus on maintaining good relationships with large employers and payers in their market to make sure they're meeting their needs. In the end, that's really the only thing they can control. When the needs of employers and payers are met, there's less incentive for them to go out and seek alternatives. Local providers must be in constant dialogue with those paying the bills—this can't be a one time or occasional occurrence.

Our hospitals should also consider how they might participate in medical travel themselves. Can they partner internationally to offer expertise or even deliver services to patients who chose to travel outside of the country for care? In other words, if you can't beat them, then join them.

Of course, the decision to partner internationally is not an easy one. Healthcare isn't a 'plug-and-play' service; just because a provider is successful here, does not mean that it can be successful everywhere.

There's also the consideration of resource allocation. Hospitals everywhere are very limited in terms of overall resources, both human and capital. Getting involved in the international market means spreading those resources even thinner. Each hospital needs to examine its own situation. Does it make sense to use scarce resources in this way? Can it afford the opportunity cost of such an investment? Can it afford not to get involved in medical travel particularly if explosive growth is expected?

MTT: A year ago I interviewed John Vitalis and Barbara Cox from Noblis. One of the areas of concern they cited related to medical travel was the issue of privacy and security of patient data. How do you feel the industry is doing in terms of addressing that concern?

CSC: In the United States, there's a huge focus on the privacy and confidentiality of patient information. However, I can't comment on the standards that exist abroad. I would like to mention one other information challenge though. Quality patient care requires continuity and goes well beyond individual episodes of care. When a patient goes abroad for a medical service, there are things that must occur both before and after. Managing continuity of care can be a challenge even in a small geographic area; a challenge that's only exacerbated when huge distances are involved. This is where good information systems come in. As patients move around the globe in search of various medical services, their medical information must flow as well. To the extent that patients develop their own personal health records (PHR), at least some bare minimum of information will be tracked and maintained. However, there will continue to be issues and barriers to truly effective information exchange across national boundaries.

MTT: Do you have any final thoughts on medical travel?
CSC: Certainly we are doing many things right in healthcare in this country. But is it affordable? By providing viable alternatives, medical travel forces U.S. providers to examine the value of their services and ensure that it is on par with other alternatives both at home and abroad. In that sense, it is a very positive force for our health care system.

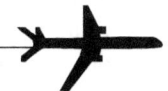

Connie Chow
Senior Vice President
MissionCare, Inc.

January 2009

Laura Carabello, publisher and managing editor, recently interviewed Connie Chow, RN, MN, NEA-BC senior vice president, MissionCare, Inc. Taipei, Taiwan.

Medical Travel Today (MTT): Tell us your background, how you became involved in health care administration, and now in the field of medical travel?
Connie Chow (CC): I was born in Taiwan, the daughter of a pilot who traveled extensively during the late 1960s and early 1970s. My family lived in Vietnam when I was seven, then I moved with my family to Thailand where I was enrolled in the International School. We then moved to Taiwan where I attended an American school. My older brother had made his way to Oklahoma, and I followed him there as a young teenager. Fortunately, I was introduced to an American family who agreed to sponsor me and lived in Oklahoma throughout high school.

I always wanted to be a nurse, so after high school, I was accepted to attend California State University's Bakersfield Nursing Program, and thanks to the encouragement of a mentor, went on to earn a Master's degree in Nursing from the University of California Los Angeles (UCLA). Following some work with various non-profit organizations, I went on to work at the for-profit Tenet Healthcare Corp. where I ran the rehabilitation unit. In 1994, I became a surveyor for the Joint Commission and just retired last spring after 14 years of active service.

Based upon my understanding of standards and quality, I was invited in 2005 to work at MissionCare in Taiwan. Although I still reside in California, I travel one to two months between Taiwan and California. Having the good fortune of being able to travel worldwide during my youth and later on as a surveyor for the Joint Commission, I was able to help our flagship hospital, Min-Sheng, form its International Health Care Department in January 2008. This is the sequence of events that led to my involvement in the global operations.

MTT: Can you provide an overview of Min Sheng Hospital and its role in providing services to Americans?
CC: Min-Sheng is a 600-bed, private general hospital, the flagship of the MissionCare Corporation, which is one of the biggest health care chains that operates seven healthcare facilities (hospitals, clinics, and long-term care) in Taiwan. The hospital was built in 2001 and equipped with state-of-the-art technologies such as high-speed CT, PACS, and minimally invasive operations rooms. Min-Sheng obtained its JCI accreditation in 2006, and is pursuing JCI disease-specific certificate on AMI-STEMI by the end of 2008. It will soon become Taiwan's first Center of Excellence in cardiac care.

MissionCare, Inc.— the corporate parent of Min-Sheng Hospital—began developing international services following the JCI accreditation, with aims to attract foreign patients from the United States and other countries for high quality and affordable health care services. Following this goal, the hospital has enhanced its services to be more English-friendly and created several mechanisms to facilitate the care delivered to foreign patients, such as obtaining contractual agreements with various global health insurances, establishing a single communication window, handling pre-approval and screening processes, care protocols, one-on-one services, and concierge services.

Currently, the hospital has some experience in serving American patients. Most of these are local expatriates who work as English teachers, engineers, or multi-national corporation staff. We also serve some American patients with emergency medical needs during their travels. For example, there was one woman who experienced serious diarrhea at the airport that caused her to miss her connecting flight for the United States. Because we are the closest hospital to the airport, she was transported here. We not only rendered proper medical care to her but also provided options for payment, and allowed her to deposit payment to our U.S. bank for her convenience.

We've also had numerous American patients travel to Taiwan for bariatric surgery. Additionally, we provided services to a patient from the United States who was seeking shoulder arthroscopy. Upon further examination of this individual, our orthopedic surgeon determined that the patient did not need the procedure.

Another trend is that we have served many Chinese Americans, some Mainland Chinese, and a few Saudi clients for their comprehensive health check-ups, with immediate intervention and treatment if the check-up uncovered abnormal findings. Most patients appreciated the convenience of getting all the screening examinations performed and most test results within six hours – a significant time savings compared with the U.S. facilities, which often require several visits, travel to different sites for examination, and long waiting periods.

MTT: Please give us your perspectives on the importance of JCI accreditation.
CC: JCI accreditation is a minimum requirement for any hospital aiming to develop international business. However, it won't guarantee the success of this business or ensure the flow of foreign patients coming to the hospital after achieving the stamp of approval. We've been approached by many global health insurance companies and medical travel agents these past few years, and the very first question they ask is if we are JCI accredited. So, as you can see, JCI accreditation has been recognized by the insurer and other intermediaries as a means to assure the hospital meets "International Quality Standards." The importance of JCI accreditation toward international healthcare is that it's currently the most recognized third-party healthcare quality accreditation authority worldwide. With JCI accreditation, the hospital has to focus its care on the patient and must continuously monitor quality indicators, assure consistent quality outcomes, continuously improve -- and never remain status quo. JCI accreditation process is equivalent to the Joint Commission accreditation process in the United States because the accreditation originated from the Joint Commission.

This year, JCI published it 3rd edition standards, and it has put emphasis and new standards on cultural diversity, physician-specific quality performance indicators, and minimizing language barriers.

MTT: What are the hospital's areas of strength and centers of excellence?
CC: Min-Sheng specializes in minimally invasive surgeries, including minimally invasive cardiac surgeries (PTCA and mini-bypass), mini-invasive varicose vein

treatment (EVLT, Sclerotherapy, and Muller's phlebectomy), mini-invasive bariatric surgeries (lab-band, bypass, gastrectomy, and gastric balloon), and mini-invasive orthopedic surgeries (spine, laminectomy), urological procedures, such as laser prostectomy, and gynecological surgeries that are performed endoscopically. In addition, we are featuring Lasik revision surgery using wave-front guided equipment, and infertility treatments with a higher-than-standard success rate. We also offer comprehensive health checkup programs that perform all screening tests within half a day in a luxury, hotel-like environment.

MTT: Is English spoken by doctors and other health professionals?
CC: Yes, English is spoken by our doctors. All doctors in Taiwan receive medical training using English textbooks. Some of our physicians have received additional trainings or fellowships in the United States and Canada. Our nurses speak simple English, and we also have some English-fluent care coordinators who are competent to assist American patients throughout the whole care process.

MTT: Can you provide a procedure-specific cost comparison?
CC: Overall, the cost of healthcare in Taiwan is one third of that in the United States.

MTT: Please describe your programs for ensuring quality and safety.
CC: We follow JCI standards regarding patient safety and quality. We stay compliant and survey-ready all the time. Taiwan also has its own accreditation processes that oversee and ensure quality. They monitor physician practices such as mortality rates, overuse of antibiotics, appropriate antibiotic use, and medication use. In addition, we have used the electronic physician order entries and automated pharmacy-dispensing machines since 2001. This process ensures medication safety. JCI is not the end all -- in reality, it is just the beginning. JCI helps organizations to reach an international level of quality standards. I feel that all hospitals should be JCI-accredited, and it should be the basic requirement for any hospital seeking to serve foreign patients.

MTT: Is Taiwan an American-friendly environment?
CC: Overall, Taiwan's living environment is safer than many other countries. The crime rate is far lower than many major cities in the United States. Street signs are bilingual and most citizens speak some English and are friendly. Shops stay open until 10 in the evening. We drive on the same side of the street, and we use the same electrical voltages. We have great public transportation to get around, and there is less traffic problems compared to other Asian countries. Food is safe and clean to eat, plus there are many American chains such as Subway, McDonald's, Kentucky Fried Chicken, Pizza Hut, and TGI Fridays, etc.

All physicians at the hospital are educated using English textbooks and many can communicate in English – the result of international travel, which makes them fluent. In fact, we provide for nurses to participate in on-site English workshops that help staff members to improve and practice speaking English.

MTT: Do you maintain contracts with US-based employers, travel coordinators, or health plans?
CC: We are signing contracts with various insurance and medical tourism companies as we speak; some of the contracts we have in place include: Aetna Global Benefits—since 2006 UnitedHealth International—since 2007 International SOS—since

2007 BridgeHealth International—2008 Cigna International Expatriate Benefit—since 2008 Companion Global Health—since 2008 Mondial Assistance—since 2008

MTT: How can Americans make arrangements to utilize your hospital?
CC: We provide English-speaking hotlines for overseas patients, as well as Web site and e-mail access. We also have two staff—one in California and one in Arizona—to answer inquiries. Most communications are e-mail based, and all e-mails receive prompt replies within 24 hours of receipt.

To contact our U.S. representatives, Ms. Fu (California): +1 626 376 5113 or Mr. Neeley (Arizona): +1 480 335 8666 http://www.missioncare.com.tw/

MTT: Why should Americans choose your hospital over other international facilities?
CC: Taiwan is the gateway toward other Southeast Asia countries such as Thailand, Singapore, Malaysia, and India. It's at least three hours of flight time closer if flying from the United States.

Taiwan's overall living environment and quality are higher than many other Southeast Asia countries, and the healthcare environment is technology-driven in many aspects, especially the development of information technology. We have computerized physician order entry and filmless PACS system. Medical information can be converted and portable, allowing patients to transport it home for better follow-up. Finally, our costs are lower than Singapore and comparable to Thailand.

Taiwan is a politically stable country, very Americanized and safe. We believe American patients will feel right at home coming to Taiwan. The global economy will drive increased patient visits here—and we are safe, quality-oriented and ready to receive them.

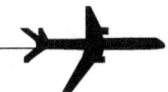

Joseph S. Barcie, M.D.
President
International Hospital Corporation

February 2009

When International Hospital Corporation (IHC) set about building hospitals in Latin America, they no doubt had some faith in the adage "build it and they will come." What they didn't know was that the "they" that would arrive wouldn't be just the local community they expected to serve but also international patients looking for an alternative to the care available in their homeland.

Medical Travel Today *recently spoke to Dr. Barcie about his role at IHC and his expectations for the organization's expanding international patients department.*

Medical Travel Today (MTT): Tell me about your role at International Hospital Corporation and what it means to be in charge of centralized services?
Jose Barcie (JB): IHC started 12 years ago with our first CIMA Hospital in Mexico. CIMA expanded operations within Mexico and Central America and later acquired the VITA hospital group in Brazil.

The CIMA hospitals in Mexico and Central America operated very independently of each other. The VITA hospitals in Brazil, however, were a well-established group before they joined our system.

I was hired by IHC to help make the hospital departments within the CIMA Hospitals operate well together as a system. I was charged with standardizing hospital services. For example, each hospital had its own departments for marketing, information technology, quality and safety, education, clinical research, and so on. These all needed to work together as a system. And that's what I did and continue to do.

MTT: You mentioned international patients. How much of your time would you say is devoted specifically to that area?
JB: Well, I'm very fortunate in that I have a very strong regional manager in Ms. Balbina Lankenau de la Garza. She came to us after working as the international patient coordinator for another company. She joined us a year ago. Because of her efforts and those of her team, I'm only devoting about 14 percent of my time to that area.

MTT: That still sounds like a good bit of your time.
JB: Yes, I suppose, but it's no longer devoted to the establishment of the department and hiring staff, but rather to development and expansion. We're constantly looking for more ways to serve our medical traveler. When I examine our competition, I see more than a few areas of concerns. We want to make sure we continue to do everything better, by constantly raising the quality and safety bar. I'm focusing a great deal on ensuring we provide the best continuum of care for all our patients, local or international.

MTT: Did you anticipate spending as much time and energy on medical travel issues as you currently do?

JB: No. Although, everyone seems to think this would be a big growth opportunity, we were focusing our primary attention on the local community we serve. Our hospitals were not developed for the purpose of attracting international patients, but soon we discovered that our hospitals were ideally located to meet the needs of those who were looking for the best and highest quality services close to home.

MTT: Earlier this year you noted that IHC first saw an increase in foreign patients five years ago. What's been the trend in terms of numbers of patients over the past year?
JB: In the past five years the number of international patients has been growing at a very steady rate without marketing and advertising. People are simply finding us through word-of-mouth. I believe this rate could be even higher if we actually spent some time marketing our services.

MTT: Are all your hospitals experiencing the same increase in international patients?
JB: Generally speaking all the hospitals are seeing the same rate of growth with regards to international patients. But, if I had to pick one as a leader, I'd say CIMA Costa Rica gets slightly more international patients. And that's probably because there are so many U.S. ex-pats living in Costa Rica who have direct communication with family and friends in the United States. I believe that if they have seen the hospital, they are a source of encouragement in terms of coming to CIMA San Jose for any treatment.

MTT: What do you have in the works in terms of marketing?
JB: We're currently evaluating several very interesting strategies. The end result is that more people will know about our attention to detail and passion for providing safe, quality healthcare at an affordable price. That's why we say "It's your safest medical care close to home ®."

MTT: Where are the majority of your foreign patients currently coming from and how has that changed, if at all, over the past year or so?
JB: At the moment the vast majority of our patients come from the United States and Canada, with a small percentage coming from other Latin American countries like Argentina, Chile, and Panama. Where patients come from hasn't changed much, but what they come for sure has. In the early years most of our international patients came for cosmetic procedures and weight control procedures. While those numbers are still holding steady, we see more and more patients coming for more complex surgeries like orthopedics, cardiology, and neurology.

MTT: Tell me a bit about the Medical Value Travel Department?
JB: In order to better serve the international patient, we established the Medical Value Travel (MVT) as the regional office for our international patient care services offered by any of our hospitals, whether they are in Costa Rica, Mexico, or Brazil. It's based out of Monterrey, Mexico, because Monterrey is one of the three most important cities in Mexico and a modern industrial and business center with a strong relationship with the United States. The office, which is available 24/7, year round, is staffed by Ms. Lankenau and her dedicated staff. All of our hospitals are in daily contact with this office.

MTT: Do you all your international patients work through that office?

JB: Yes. We found that it's less stressful for the typical patient to contact us there. The MVT team then works to find the appropriate physician and facility in our system that matches their needs, based on both specialty and proximity.

MTT: What does the creation of a Medical Value Travel department do to your relationship with other medical travel facilitators? Do you still partner with them?

JB: Yes. We firmly believe that having MVT benefits the medical travel facilitator by providing a central point of contact. They no longer have to contact so many different hospitals or doctors; it's a one-stop shop for the facilitator. However, we're very slow to partner with facilitators. Right now sitting at my desk I have 18 contracts for review from medical facilitators.

The truth is that because there are no barriers to entry, anyone can become a medical travel facilitator. We feel it's necessary to do a very thorough background check of prospective partners for the sake of the medical traveler. We can afford to be choosy. People are eager to work with us because not only are we the largest Pan-Latin American hospital group but we stand by our word to provide the safest medical care close to home.

And, I encourage anyone considering traveling abroad to make sure they do their homework, too. Don't just compare prices. Healthcare in foreign countries is not a commodity.

MTT: In addition to creating the MVT department this year in Monterrey, Mexico, specifically for international patients pre- and post-treatment needs, what other plans are currently in the works or being discussed to continue addressing the needs of this market?

JB: The decision to create the MVT department came about because of our desire to provide international patients with a complete service model with continuity of care, before, during, and after having their procedure. Towards that end we offer our patients continued support from all our staff and doctors before they arrive, during their stay, after discharge, while convalescing, and even after they return home.

MTT: Since we're at the start of a New Year, what product or service related to medical travel that doesn't exist today do you think might exist next year at this time?

JB: Maybe additional growth in the post-op care area. We would like to see more U.S. physicians and nurses get involved in this very young market.

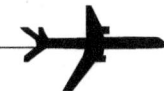

Jason Hwang, M.D., MBA
Senior Strategist
Healthcare Practice at Innosight, LLC

April 2009

Jason Hwang, M.D., M.B.A. is an internal medicine physician and senior strategist for the Healthcare Practice at Innosight LLC, an innovation and strategy consulting firm. He also co-founded and serves as the executive director of Healthcare at Innosight Institute, a non-profit social innovation think tank. Together with Professor Clayton M. Christensen of Harvard Business School and the late Jerome H. Grossman of Harvard Kennedy School of Government, he is co-author of The Innovator's Prescription: A Disruptive Solution for Health Care *(McGraw-Hill, January 2009).*

Previously, Dr. Hwang taught as chief resident and clinical instructor at the University of California, Irvine, where he received multiple recognitions for his clinical work. He has also served as a clinician with the Southern California Kaiser Permanente Medical Group and the Department of Veterans Affairs Medical Center in Long Beach, California. Dr. Hwang received his B.S. and M.D. from the University of Michigan and his M.B.A. from Harvard Business School.

Medical Travel Today (MTT): How does medical travel impact the social fabric of Americans?
Jason Hwang (JH): Our view of medical travel is that it is a long-term trend that has been developing for over a century. Today, travel is easier, and people are willing and able to go great distances—not simply to the next town – for better care.

As a business concept, medical travel destinations should be focused on quality through specialization, not simply lower cost. Individuals need to be incented to travel, and ultimately both quality and cost will provide the impetus to travel for medical care. Specialization is not really a new concept, but eventually it will become the primary reason that people will travel for care. The question is: will foreign hospitals do a better job than U.S. institutions? This remains to be seen.

MTT: Should hospitals be focusing on achieving quality or efficiency – or both?
JH: Quality is the buzzword in the industry, but it means different things to different audiences. Quality needs to be defined in a way that is relevant to the "job" that a patient is "hiring" a hospital to do, with benchmarks set and communicated to patients so that they can arrive at their own conclusions.

To achieve quality in any setting, hospitals need to focus on a particular job or specialty to do it well – and do it efficiently. By focusing on a particular area, such as cardiac or orthopedic care, some hospitals can choose to deliver a full continuum of care from pre-op to post-op and rehab…and everything in between, in a truly integrated manner that delivers high value. Other hospitals can focus simply on a select procedure, such as valve replacement or hip resurfacing, provided that the patient's job-to-be-done is simply to repair a known problem.

With this specialized attention and integration of services surrounding the delivery of care, hospitals will achieve higher quality while delivering more value. When you focus on a particular job, you not only become more proficient, you also become more cost-effective.

MTT: What other suggestions do you have for hospitals to attract patients?
JH: Many institutions will have to change their operations in order to make this happen. Creating a more customer-friendly environment requires a retail mentality. Transparency in pricing is imperative – along with information and decision tools that allow patients to make an informed choice. This is especially true for the increasing number of patients using Health Savings Accounts, where they are motivated to spend wisely.

The bottom line is that it is no longer acceptable to embrace the philosophy, "Build it and they will come." Patients need to perceive value and purchase with confidence, and hospitals need to realize that they are no longer competing locally, but globally.

MTT: Can you cite some examples of hospitals that have done a good job in communicating value?
JH: The Shouldice Hospital in Ontario, Canada, is a center of excellence for the repair of abdominal wall hernias. Within this specialty, Shouldice has become a world-class leader, attracting significant numbers of patients from the United States and worldwide.

As an example of the benefits of focus, Shouldice's stairwells are all comprised of half-steps to make it easier for hernia patients to ambulate following surgery. Specialized facilities can take these thoughts into consideration and create focused environments that completely satisfy their patients' needs. The Coxa Hospital for Joint Replacement in Tampere, Finland, by virtue of doing nothing other than endoprosthetic surgeries, achieves far lower complication rates than for similar surgeries performed at general hospitals (0.1 percent vs. 10-12 percent).

While Bumrungrad Hospital in Bangkok has excellent marketing, it is basically a "rejuvenated" U.S. model of a general hospital with amenities and upgrades. They can deliver lower pricing because of lower wage scales, but this is only a temporary advantage that is not sustainable. What is sustainable is a specialty focus that leads to quality and efficiency—that's ultimately what will get people to travel.

MTT: Do you foresee increased traction for medical travel among employers, health plans and other payers?
JH: Insurance companies and health plans are in a somewhat adversarial relationship with their customers. While they strive to introduce cost-saving initiatives such as medical travel, they do not want to be perceived as sacrificing quality for the sake of higher profits.

However, we believe that by offering access to specialty hospitals that do in fact produce higher quality, payers and other stakeholders can achieve this delicate balance. This is particularly relevant to employers seeking cost savings but who are unwilling to bend on the delivery of quality, focused care.

MTT: Are patients informed and equipped to make their own decisions regarding optimal destinations for medical travel?

JH: As in any other market, some people will need help while others can do it on their own. There are now web-based tools and multiple portals that are readily accessed, as well as telephone connectivity to knowledgeable professionals. Personal financial advisors can also assist when health savings accounts are involved.

In addition, both domestic and international systems must make quality measures available for aggregation and comparison by trustworthy, transparent third parties. There must be consumer-friendly information that is relevant to individual requirements.

MTT: Going forward, will the opportunity to visit and tour a foreign country be important to medical travelers?
JH: Foreign governments and tourist boards like to think so, but for most patients this is an added bonus and secondary to the core "job." All else being equal, the opportunity to travel can be an enticement, but we believe that few patients, provided with the necessary information and guidance, would base their treatment decision on anything other than the ability to receive affordable, quality care.

MTT: What is your advice to U.S.-domestic hospitals?
JH: Focus! Look at the Mayo Clinic as an example of a hospital that recognizes the importance of focusing on patients by creating departments that address individual conditions. There's no reason a U.S. hospital can't achieve the same principles of quality and efficiency through focus that we advocate for foreign hospitals seeking to build a medical tourism business. Whenever possible, hospitals need to assemble multi-disciplinary teams centered on specific conditions and procedures, and stop bouncing patients from doctor to doctor. This will reduce a lot of the overhead costs and poor quality that result from the way our general hospitals are currently structured.

Another strategic imperative is information transparency and publishing data that are appropriate and relevant for patients to evaluate and compare. Otherwise, patients will fall into the trap of simply basing their health decisions on cost, and that would be to everyone's detriment.

MTT: Will it be possible for domestic hospitals to reduce salaries/wages and lower the cost of care?
JH: Yes, but only if they're willing to disrupt themselves with new business models of care delivery, such as incorporating nurses, physician assistants, or technicians to provide more care. This is one of the reasons why retail clinics will be successful – the combination of low-cost venues of care and different providers of care results in an affordable and accessible means of managing simple medical problems. In contrast, it would be a mistake to reduce costs simply by cutting salaries and fees. Forcing high-cost professionals to somehow become more efficient by reducing payment will only lead to dissatisfaction across the board.

MTT: What is the bottom line to motivating patients to pursue medical travel options?
JH: When people are armed with information and incentives to travel, and when large employers empower their workforces with decision-making capabilities, the industry will grow. Much of the expansion will rely upon hospitals releasing their data and employers putting incentives in place via portable health savings accounts and shared savings programs.

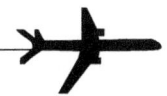

Arnon Krongrad, M.D.
Chief Executive Officer
Mobile Surgery International

May 2009

Earlier this year Medical Surgery International (MSI) treated its first patient for prostate cancer. On the surface this may not sound like big news, but the premise and the logistics of how the case was managed are actually quite noteworthy.

Headed by Arnon Krongrad, M.D., MSI flew both the patient and surgical team to a selected facility in Trinidad for the procedure. Funded by the patient, this approach allowed the patient to receive the specific surgical procedure he needed from a well-respected surgeon in a facility pre-approved by the surgeon -- all at a cost the patient could afford.

"Recent years have seen the development of a 'medical tourism' trend in which patients travel to overseas medical centers for certain types of surgical procedures at low cost," states Dr. Krongrad. "However, we believe that this particular operation in Trinidad may represent the beginning of a new trend -- in which patient and surgeon agree to 'meet' at a mutually acceptable location for cost effective, high quality surgical procedures."

Medical Travel Today *recently spoke to Dr. Krongrad to learn how this new approach evolved and about the advantages it offers patients, payers, and physicians.*

Medical Travel Today (MTT): Tell me a bit about what inspired you to launch Mobile Surgery International?
Arnon Krongrad (AK): All my life I have been surrounded by healthcare. My father was a doctor and my mother was a nurse. One of my earliest memories is of going with my father on a house call to treat a man with chest pain. Later, while in med school, I worked in a clinic in Kenya. While I was there I saw dentists flying in to provide care. And really, that was just another kind of house call.

In part, the inspiration for Mobile Surgery International (MSI) stems from those memories and the spirit of the house call. MSI strives to provide that same level of service: the treatment choice the patient needs in the location that makes the most sense for the procedure being performed.

Of course the needs of patients today are different from when my father was practicing. It's no longer about just addressing a medical issue. Today the focus is largely on cost and quality.

By taking patients abroad for care and traveling with them, the patient has the assurance – and comfort – of getting a doctor they are familiar with and the knowledge that the doctor is operating in a facility that, without question, has the technology that's needed to perform the procedure. They know this because the surgeon has selected the facility, rather than the facility having been selected by a travel coordinator who may or may not know about the proper equipment for the given procedure. In that sense, Mobile Surgery International offers surgeon-driven health travel.

Let me also add that at The Krongrad Institute in Florida, we've been treating patients from abroad for the past 10 years. We see patients from Japan, Chile ... really from all over. So the whole idea of medical travel was not new to us. What MSI brings to the equation is the idea of seeking out specific facilities or hospitals for specific procedures. Honestly, a doctor doesn't care if a facility is on a tropical island or on the moon. What they care about is that it has the right equipment and standards of care for the patient. That's where we put our focus. We're prepared to consider every permutation that will provide choice, quality, and cost containment.

MTT: How did you come to develop a working relationship with U.S. Risk Underwriters?
AK: When we were preparing to launch MSI we looked for insurance products that help limit risk. We looked at a number of products including health travel products. One product didn't strike us as credible and another was from a well-known company but it excluded cancer surgery. That presented a problem for the type of patients we treat. Then we found U.S. Risk Underwriters. They have a product that they sell directly to patients that covers their risks and cancer.

Obviously there's a wonderful synergy between what each of us provides. But let me be clear: we have no financial relationship with U.S. Risk Underwriters, Inc. There's no benefit to us if a patient chooses their policy. But, as with all products or services we think might be useful to our clients, we certainly tell them about it.

The truth is, when someone is dealing with a medical issue, especially one like cancer, they've got enough of a burden to deal with. So if we can recommend insurance coverage, accommodation, or other services that alleviate some of the burden, we do it.

MTT: How did you decide to choose Trinidad as a medical destination?
AK: We didn't select Trinidad. We selected an operating room. In medical travel there's this general notion that you select a location, but to a doctor the tourist attractions are immaterial. We select by specific equipment we need for the procedure. In this case we selected the high definition flat panel video monitor. We complemented it with such preferred and portable gizmos as a 24 French grooved urethral sound and a voice-controlled robot.

I spent and continue to spend a lot of time visiting hospitals. In the same way that the Joint Commission will visit a facility and look at infection rates and the cleanliness of the lobby, a surgeon visits a facility but looks at different things. In my visits I'm looking to see specific equipment. By introducing surgical subject authority into medical travel you introduce a different perspective on what's important. Again, if you want quality surgery, you don't care where it is. You care about who is performing it and in what operating setting. And to be honest, if you want to get serious about cost containment in healthcare, you need to involve surgeons -- not administrators -- in these choices.

While the hospital we selected has the right stuff, one of its most appealing aspects is that an anesthesiologist runs it. For a surgeon, having a conversation with people who have been to an operating room just makes the whole discussion very efficient and productive. You're both coming at the topic from the same vantage point, and it's extremely helpful in surgical program development. The people at our Trinidad facility understand the issues and needs and can address them precisely without adding on unnecessary items or expenses.

MTT: Are you operating in other locations or looking to do so?

AK: The short answer is yes. The long answer is that there are all kinds of considerations that have to be addressed before you can access the advantages of flexible surgery options. For example, there's the fact that people from Jamaica would in some cases prefer to go to Miami than to Trinidad for surgery. Some of what makes a location work or not work is personal and cultural preference.

MSI is certainly looking at other host facilities to address this issue and to help patients and regional payers better work with us. Our priority is a host hospital in a Latin country. We have recently gotten feelers from the Ukraine and from Israel. I'm not surprised. For the hospitals, here and abroad, Mobile Surgery International represents elimination of the learning curve, reduction in capital expenditure, and acceleration of time to market.

MTT: Thus far the procedures you've performed abroad have been related to prostate cancer. Do you intend to provide other types of procedures?

AK: Obviously prostate surgery is my area of personal practice expertise so that's been the initial focus. (Editor's Note: Dr. Krongrad pioneered the use of laparoscopic radical prostatectomy in the United States.)

However, MSI is now in the process of developing a network of highly specialized surgeons. Among others, we're looking at adding surgeons with cardiac, colorectal, and orthopedic expertise, as quickly as possible.

The model works so well for prostate surgery that the idea of opening up to other areas isn't intimidating to me. It's also important to note that most Americans aren't going abroad for cancer surgery. Plastic surgery and orthopedics are still the biggest draws. But I believe that by bringing in specialists you alleviate the fear and notion that you can't get quality care abroad. It also works for the host hospitals, as they are now able to add an area of expertise to their roster that they didn't have before.

MTT: How has the recruiting effort been going? Are doctors interested?

AK: Yes, the doctors are interested. The doctors like being doctors. They like taking care of people and they like operating. And they get how this model makes sense. It's largely physician driven. Just as the doctors get it, the payers are starting to get it, too.

MTT: How has your decision to travel abroad to perform procedures affected your working relationships with hospitals here in the United States?

AK: Mobile Surgery International aims to preserve choice and quality for the patient. In the case of this specific patient, the only way to preserve choice was to go to Trinidad. Why? Because he was uninsured, had little money, and he could not find an affordable choice at home. Given our aims, we went to Trinidad. However, in most cases we bring patients to the United States, including from Trinidad.

The model MSI is developing offers domestic hospitals and hospital chains the same benefits as it provided for the hospital in Trinidad: flattening of learning curves, reduction in cost, and acceleration of time to market. This means that our model can help many domestic hospitals get the same quality and choice with cost containment.

More specifically, MSI's visibility has been very good for the domestic hospital at which we are headquartered. Why? Because it has resulted in new inquiries from domestic and foreign payers. For example, this morning we finalized agreements with an Israeli payer that wants to send new patients to us in Miami and an American third party administrator that wants access to our Aventura and Trinidad options. These payers approached us because of MSI's special subject expertise and its emphasis on quality. They approached us now because our work in the field exposed them to what we do.

We have always brought in patients from abroad. Since setting up MSI, our American base has been referring patients from such new and varied sources as Ukraine, Curacao, and New Zealand. Why? Because patients and payers alike appreciate choice and quality. They seek it in Trinidad and they seek it in Miami. Using surgical subject expertise, MSI is developing an operational model and a culture of service that will enable them to receive choice and quality with cost containment whenever applicable.

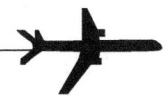

Joseph M. Heyman, M.D.
Past Chair, Board of Trustees
American Medical Association

June 2009

Editor's Note: *When President Obama delivered his remarks on healthcare reform at the American Medical Association (AMA) meeting in June, he began by thanking Dr. Joseph Heyman, then Chair of the AMA's Board of Trustees.*

Dr. Heyman has been involved in organized medicine since joining the Massachusetts Medical Society (MMS) in 1973. He joined the AMA in 1980 and has been a member of the Massachusetts delegation to the AMA since 1987. He was a member of the AMA Council on Medical Service, serving on its executive committee (1997–2000) and as its Chair (2000–2001). During his tenure on the council, Dr. Heyman helped develop AMA policy on health insurance reform, pharmaceutical industry spending in the United States, and hospital mergers.

Medical Travel Today *recently put some questions to Dr. Heyman regarding the up- and downsides of medical travel and his thoughts on how the proposed reform measures might impact the industry.*

Medical Travel Today **(MTT): Can you share with us your thoughts on the up- and downsides of medical travel for both consumers and physicians?**
Paul Heyman (PH): We believe patients should have choice in healthcare. That includes being able to choose medical travel. We want our patients to take an active role in their healthcare decision-making, and we believe that choosing from whom and where to receive healthcare is not a decision that should be arrived at lightly. Whether care is provided in the United States or abroad, it's important for patients to be confident in the qualifications of the physician providing their care, as well as the safety standards of the hospital or clinic where the care will be given.

The risks of seeking care outside the United States can be significant. Fewer international hospitals meet the same quality standards imposed by accrediting organizations like Joint Commission International, as opposed to those in the United States. Patients may have a hard time trying to assess the qualifications of the physician and facility providing the care. In some countries there may be no legal recourse for poor outcomes. Seeking healthcare overseas, particularly with long flights following surgery, carries an increased risk of developing complications, such as blood clots, swelling, and infection.

MTT: Pre- and post-op care is one of the biggest concerns physicians have about medical travel. What advice might you share with physicians regarding addressing the issue with patients?
PH: It's essential that patients going abroad for care have a physician and follow-up care plan in place prior to treatment to ensure that they receive the proper follow-up and lessen the risk for complications when they return home.

MTT: What can U.S. physicians do in order to be more competitive with non-domestic providers?

PH: A strong patient-physician relationship is incredibly important, and we want our patients to be comfortable talking to us about their medical concerns and decisions. While a cheaper price has often been sighted as one of the main reasons Americans go overseas for care, it is important that price not be the only factor in determining where and from whom to receive medical treatment.

MTT: Clearly the goal of the proposed reform measures is to make health-care more affordable and accessible to all Americans. As one in the field, what do you think is a realistic timeline for seeing meaningful change and how dramatic might it truly be? That is, will the cost of a hip replacement in the United States be competitive with the cost of one in India?

PH: We expect health reform to happen this year. We are committed to achieving reform that ensures all Americans have affordable, high-quality health coverage and can get the best value from healthcare spending.

The American Medical Association has guidelines for choosing international travel. They are as follows:

H-450.937 Medical Care Outside the United States

Our AMA advocates that employers, insurance companies, and other entities that facilitate or incentivize medical care outside the United States adhere to the following principles:

1. Medical care outside of the United States must be voluntary.
2. Financial incentives to travel outside the United States for medical care should not inappropriately limit the diagnostic and therapeutic alternatives that are offered to patients or restrict treatment or referral options.
3. Patients should only be referred for medical care to institutions that have been accredited by recognized international accrediting bodies (e.g., the Joint Commission International or the International Society for Quality in Health Care).
4. Prior to travel, local follow-up care should be coordinated and financing should be arranged to ensure continuity of care when patients return from medical care outside the United States.
5. Coverage for travel outside the United States for medical care must include the costs of necessary follow-up care upon return to the United States.
6. Patients should be informed of their rights and legal recourse prior to agreeing to travel outside the United States for medical care.
7. Access to physician licensing and outcome data, as well as facility accreditation and outcomes data, should be arranged for patients seeking medical care outside the United States.
8. The transfer of patient medical records to and from facilities outside the United States should be consistent with the Health Insurance Portability and Accountability Act (HIPAA) guidelines.
9. Patients choosing to travel outside the United States for medical care should be provided with information about the potential risks of combining surgical procedures with long flights and vacation activities (CMS Rep. 1, A-08)

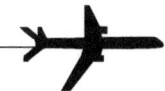

John C. Goodman
President & Chief Executive Officer
National Center for Policy Analysis

June 2009

Editor's Note: *Readers are no doubt familiar with John C. Goodman, president and CEO of the National Center for Policy Analysis (NCPA). Often referred to as the "Father of Health Savings Accounts," Goodman also maintains a health policy blog where pro-free enterprise, private sector solutions to health care problems are routinely examined and debated by top health policy.*

In light of the recently proposed health reforms, Medical Travel Today *decided to catch up with Goodman and find out what he and his colleagues think of the proposed reforms and how they may or may not influence domestic and foreign medical travel.*

***Medical Travel Today* (MTT): Thank you for your time today and your willingness to discuss the future of medical travel.**
John Goodman (JG): It's my pleasure. If I may, I'd like to suggest we start this interview by asking the question, "Why would anyone go outside the United States for healthcare?"

MTT: By all means, proceed.
JG: In the United States, healthcare costs are growing at twice the rate of our income. It's been this way for the past 40 years and there are no signs of abatement.

When any major expenditure grows at twice the rate of the consumer's income, the consumer gets squeezed. In the United States we have no price competition for healthcare. And that's because you tend to have competition on price only when there's no third-party payer. Interestingly, if hospitals and physicians do not compete on price, they don't compete on quality either. So in order for U.S. citizens to get the full benefit of competition, they have to leave the country.

MTT: As you point out, the U.S. system is built around a third-party payer. Given that, is there anything a U.S. provider can do to compete?
JG: I believe there is, but it involves more than a new model. It involves a new mind set in the way we approach care. I believe that in order to keep patients here, we have to have facilities that are willing to post their prices and are willing to compete on price.

The successful facilities internationally are the ones that are willing to quote package prices and make those prices truly transparent to customers.

As deductibles rise and co-pays rise, what we're seeing is that patients and insurance companies, who were once adversaries, now find themselves on the same team -- a team that's looking to find the best price and quality options for care.

What we're going to see is insurers and employers encouraging patients to travel (both within the country and out of the country) for lower-priced, higher-quality care. The resulting savings are going to be shared by the insurers and employers with the patients. That type of model is going to force U.S. facilities to compete in a different way if they are going to stay in business.

MTT: Which facilities in the United States are best prepared to deal with this kind of competition?
JG: The ones that are already involved in treating foreign patients. Right now there are about 50 major U.S. hospitals actively marketing in Latin America to recruit patients. They're already competing in an international marketplace and many are doing it with a package price structure. They are doing the things they need to do to compete effectively on quality and price in a global market.

MTT: How do you move from an environment where there's no price competition to one where there is?
JG: Well, first you have to look at what is preventing U.S. healthcare from becoming competitive, the way hospitals in Thailand, India, or Singapore are competing.

The difference is that we have a lot of unwise public policies that suppress normal market forces. As a result, for a typical doctor or hospital there is no such thing as a real price. When Secretary of Health and Human Services Mike Leavitt last year spoke of the need for providers to post prices, what he didn't say is there are no prices, there are only reimbursement rates. In truth, we're very far away from a real market. What needs to happen are economic, cultural, and legal changes.

First, if providers are going to compete on price and quality, everyone needs to change what he or she is doing. And no one is going to change unless there are economic incentives to do so.

Second, doctors and hospitals need to change how they think about the product of healthcare. Most doctors today don't think of themselves as competing in a marketplace. In the future they will need to. Finally, we need to repeal laws that prevent competition. We really don't need to look much further than surgi-centers, urgent care centers, and walk-in clinics for a working model of how this can be done. Competition can work. All of these products developed outside the third-party system and they work for both the patient and the provider.

MTT: Given how slowly things tend to move when it comes to changing healthcare regulations and laws, what's the downside of the status quo?
JG: I think the flow of patients across the border will grow and it will grow fast. All over Latin America there are medical facilities that could be competing for U.S. patients. They are not aggressively marketing and competing for U.S. patients right now but they could.

Currently there are wealthy people who willingly travel to the Cooper Clinic in Dallas and to other facilities around the country for what I call a super-duper check-up. It's becoming a very common experience.

However, once a person commits to climbing on a plane for care, he can go anywhere to receive it. He might go to Guatemala City instead of Dallas and obtain the same quality of care for a fraction of the cost. When you start to think competitively about healthcare, you have to consider all the places that a plane might fly to.

The international market place has the potential to become one of the strongest agents of change in the way medicine is practiced in the United States.

I think Medicare does not cover medical care outside the country. If the government had any sense, they'd change that. You could save a lot of money if you encouraged seniors, your largest consumers of care, to get care abroad. This is a difficult issue for politicians to talk about. They all have doctors and hospitals as constituents, as well as patients.

I think the question is: what's the right public policy within the United States? What's the right way to encourage a competitive market for healthcare?

One way to do that is to open up the market for, say, Medicare patients. I think Medicare ought to pay walk-in clinics' market rates, not Medicare rates. Seniors aren't as desirable at Medicare rates to walk-ins or to urgent care clinics and surgicenters, for that matter. Medicare should be willing to pay the market rates, since those are still lower than what they'll have to pay at traditional facilities. Plus, you'd get more seniors seeking care earlier and that will ultimately keep all costs down.

We also need to change the tax laws to make it as easy as possible for patients to self-insure and manage more of their own healthcare dollars. If you make patients a partner in decisions you'll change their behavior and, in turn, force doctors to compete on price. That's the direction we should be heading.

MTT: What's your opinion of the recent proposals from the White House?
JG: The approach being taken by the Obama administration is the wrong approach. They think they can change the practice of medicine urging providers to produce higher quality, lower cost care from the demand side of the market. Yet they can't point to single example of that happening. Anywhere.

All the examples of lowering healthcare costs and increasing quality come from supply side. It was doctors and entrepreneurs who created those models. We need to find new ways to encourage the supply side of the market to come up with more of those approaches. The current system is so inefficient and wasteful that providers should be able to find innumerable improvements if allowed to do so.

We need more deregulation, not more regulation. We need to make it as easy as possible for hospitals and doctors to repackage and deliver their products in ways that decrease cost and increase quality of care. Right now, their hands are often tied by regulations. Hospitals in India and Thailand can repackage their products on a moment's notice. If we want to compete, providers have to have that same freedom and flexibility here.

MTT: You've talked about the constraints placed on U.S. facilities growing medical tourism. Are there any political constraints operating in other parts of the world?
JT: One thing I think that holds back medical tourism in other countries is the politically unpalatable result of having first world patients in a foreign country getting a level care that most of its own citizens cannot afford. That can certainly constrain growth.

One place where I don't see that as an issue is Latin America where almost everywhere there's a free healthcare system—but one that is not very good. So they are used to people who can afford better care going outside the free system and buying private care. In Canada or Britain when a Member of Parliament checks into a first-class private hospital it's scandalous. In Latin America that's considered perfectly normal.

Beyond that, I don't see too many obstacles—certainly none of the magnitude we face here at home—to other countries really competing on a world level. We just need to make sure we get there, too.

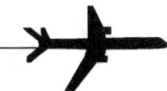

Grace-Marie Turner
President
The Galen Institute, Inc.

August 2009

The Galen Institute, Inc., is a not-for-profit, free market research organization devoted exclusively to health policy. It was founded in 1995 to promote a more informed public debate over individual freedom, consumer choice, competition, and diversity in the health sector. Galen Institute president Grace-Marie Turner recently testified before a hearing of the U.S. Senate Commerce, Science, and Transportation Committee focused on competition in the healthcare marketplace.

She said health reform legislation should "build on the innovative ideas in the private sector where improvements in the delivery and financing of healthcare, transparency, and consumer choice are working."

Medical Travel Today *spoke with her about how medical travel might fit into the vision of innovation.*

***Medical Travel Today* (MTT): During your Senate testimony you spoke of the need for innovation in healthcare delivery. How might medical travel – domestic or foreign – fit into this concept?**
Grace-Marie Turner (GMT): Many of the problems that the United States is facing involving cost, quality, and access to healthcare could be addressed by encouraging more competition and empowering consumers to have greater control over decisions involving their care and coverage.

More competition in the health sector will lead to more choices for patients. Patients should be able to make decisions, in consultation with their physicians, about where they want to go for their healthcare. That also means they should be able to decide if they want to stay in the United States or go abroad for their medical care.

I had a chance to visit a medical facility in Guatemala in April. I toured a beautiful hospital with well-trained physicians working in a state-of-the-art facility that provides care at a fraction of the charges of U.S. hospitals. There are numerous facilities of this caliber, but most of them are not yet actively marketing to U.S. patients. In the case of Guatemala, most of their patients are people from Central America who want faster access to better quality care than they could get through their public healthcare systems. Facilities like the one in Guatemala and elsewhere should be on American patients' radar as an option for care. While patients need to weigh risks against any costs savings, by all means, the government should not get in their way.

MTT: What's your opposition to government involvement?
GMT: People need more control over their healthcare resources, not less. I'm opposed to centralized government control over healthcare decisions because, among many other problems, this limits consumer's options. Consumers should be able to choose the private health insurance that best suits them and their budgets, and people should be able to go where they want for care.

The issue of transparency is hugely important, and it's one of the biggest problems with the current domestic system. Right now, most consumers know what the amount of their insurance co payment is, but they have little or no information about the total cost of their health insurance or an episode of medical care. As a result, they are not able to make informed decisions about seeking the best care affordably.

The medical travel model allows consumers to see more of the real cost of their treatment. If they can see the actual difference in pricing, not just their co-pays, they start to pay attention. It's an approach that certainly deserves more attention.

MTT: Are we moving toward that?
GMT: I frankly don't see us moving toward transparency with any of the proposals put forth by the Obama administration and Congress today. The current legislation would continue the shell game in which everyone is under the illusion that someone else is paying for their health insurance and healthcare.

What we need is innovation that offers patients more control over choices and more transparency of pricing. That would be a big step toward achieving the goals of health reform to make healthcare and health coverage more affordable and accessible. The legislation before Congress today is based upon a belief that government can make better decisions about healthcare than patients. But the best consumer choices are informed choices. More information about more affordable choices in a more competitive environment would be very beneficial to patients.

MTT: Has the option of medical travel been a part of the debate?
GMT: Medical travel so far has not been part of the health reform debate in Washington. I've attended a number of conferences where I have learned about medical tourism and its possibilities. But the longer it stays off the radar screen of politicians, the better.

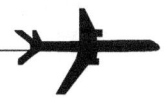

Trude Bennett
Associate Professor
University of North Carolina
Gillings School of Global Public Health

August 2009

Editor's Note: *Trude Bennett is an associate professor at the University of North Carolina's Gillings School of Global Public Health. In 2008 she spent a significant amount of time in Southeast Asia studying the effects of medical tourism on local economies and societies.*

As a health policy researcher and interested observer of transnational health services in Southeast Asia, I am frequently asked by friends and colleagues to define the term "medical tourism." Knowing that medical tourism has multiple meanings depending on context, constituency, and stakeholder, I have tried to clarify my perspective on what does and does not constitute medical tourism. My basic explanation would be the marketing of health services in receiving countries to visitors from sending countries who are traveling specifically for the purpose of seeking medical care, as well as expatriate workers living in the receiving nations. Receiving countries are usually low- or middle-income; medical travelers are usually from wealthier countries or from the upper classes of poor countries.

My specific interest is the impact of medical tourism on access to and quality of health care for local residents in countries offering foreigners "First World medical services at Third World prices." Is this truly a "win-win" situation with unalloyed benefits for all? Some enthusiasts view healthcare as a global commodity or a form of international outsourcing; they argue for the economic rationality of shuttling patients around the globe for delivery of medical goods and services. In contrast, I see medical tourism as the "third tier" of health services, a kind of ultra-privatized care that may exacerbate the differences between public and private sectors.

Close examination of the dynamics of medical tourism, including potential benefits and harms to societies at different levels of social and economic development, is essential for ethical development of the industry. Looking beyond the individual level does transnational healthcare offer useful models or does it simply blunt the impetus for health reform in the United States and elsewhere? Can medical tourism help remedy the current economic crisis in low- and middle-income countries struggling with plunging foreign investment and disadvantageous trade balances? And how can the potential benefits be realized?

The Asian Financial Crisis of 1997 resulted in an epidemic of empty beds in newly constructed private hospitals in Thailand and Malaysia. Recognizing the profitability of the international healthcare market, companies recruited foreign patients to fill those beds and consume a range of associated services. The relative equity and fluidity between the private and public health sectors in these countries allowed economically stressed middle-class Thais and Malaysians to shift back to public facilities without sacrificing quality of care. When private care became unaffordable, patients were willing to tolerate longer queues and greater inconvenience. Meanwhile, new clients from the United States and other countries discovered the advantages of longer stays at hospitals and rehabilitation centers: more attentive care and skilled treatment by well-trained providers at affordable cost.

Medical tourism sometimes, but not always, involves cosmetic surgery or elective treatments rarely covered under health insurance policies. In the United States and other countries struggling with containment of healthcare costs, medical necessity is becoming much harder to prove (to justify coverage) even under extreme circumstances. Quite often, medical tourism presents an option for un- or underinsured persons from industrialized countries seeking treatment of conditions that are life-threatening or compromise quality of life. For example, heart valve replacement or advanced cancer treatment may be unattainable for someone without private or public health insurance in the United States and prohibitively expensive for others with high deductibles and co-payments on their policies. International services offer an alternative to medical risk, prolonged suffering, and severe debt burden or possible bankruptcy. Thus the notion of medical tourism cannot be reduced to frivolous globetrotting by wealthy Westerners seeking sun, fun, and glamour. Neither can it be posed as a solution to the U.S. healthcare crisis. One of every three people under 65 in the United States lacked any form of health insurance for some part of 2007-2008, affecting all age, racial, ethnic, and income groups. Eighty percent of the uninsured were members of working families and 70 percent lived in households with at least one person employed full-time. The Institute of Medicine has estimated that lack of health insurance leads to 18,000 preventable deaths every year in the United States. Attractive as excellent and affordable healthcare in India or Thailand may be to some Americans, it is neither feasible nor desirable to address the huge gaps for medically underserved by sending them abroad. Most people are rooted in daily family and community obligations; the majorities of Americans do not own passports and are not likely to travel 10,000 miles or more at a time of anxiety and discomfort. Medical tourism also represents an escalation of our huge carbon footprint and is subject to unexpected travel restrictions caused by epidemics, conflict, or threats of disruptions. Regional healthcare consortia may make sense for small contiguous nations, but surely the United States can extend a full range of services within its vast borders.

Some medical technologies are better developed and have been more quickly approved outside the United States, making treatment options abroad more expansive. In Southeast Asia patients have access to stem cell treatments not available in the United States due to ideological constraints on research in the past eight years. Even with changes under the new Administration, we have a lot of catching up to do. Such therapies can obviate the need for surgery and save both excessive cost and risk. The utilization of nonsurgical stem cell treatments in other countries offers lessons for the United States but cannot substitute for medical progress at home. Similarly, the lack of cost inflation due to uncontrolled liability insurance rates in other countries is a lesson in non-defensive medicine that should be heeded. While accountability may not be ironclad or perfect in the context of medical tourism, non-litigious strategies for mediating conflicts about medical outcomes are necessary for the functioning of the U.S. healthcare system. Medical tourism is not necessarily an economic boon to the receiving countries, nor does it necessarily benefit local residents and guarantee them the same quality of care offered to foreigners. National economic development often increases social inequalities, and examples abound of the detrimental health effects of social disparities in income, environment, and access to resources. Medical tourism may actually drive up the cost of private care for local residents, as well as deprive patients in the public sector of providers trained at government expense.

Medical tourism as a stimulus to "internal brain drain" is clearly illustrated in Thailand and Malaysia. Both the Thai and Malaysian governments are boosting medical tourism through global advertising, tax incentives, and support for training of medical personnel in local institutions and specialty fellowships abroad. When Thailand instituted policies to promote investment in private hospitals, the exodus of doctors from government employment shot to 30 percent in 1997 (from 8 percent in 1994).

Twenty percent of Malaysia's hospital beds -- but 54 percent of the country's doctors --can be found in private hospitals. Chronic understaffing of nurses and doctors in Malaysia's public facilities -- whose salaries are at least three to four times lower than their counterparts in the private sector -- will ultimately erode the quality of healthcare. Furthermore, the three-year national service requirement for all Malaysian physicians is being challenged. Those who have been practicing abroad are being lured back with promises of national service waivers. Malaysian health advocates are raising concerns that such policies may result in a lack of senior specialists to train medical students and trainees in public hospitals.

Bookman and Bookman (2007) introduced the notion of medical tourism both "crowding out" and "crowding in" public health. The profitability of medical tourism tends to "crowd out" public health, with government resources (land, financial subsidies, tax breaks) diverted to private facilities with high technology, while public health services and primary care are allowed to languish. The World Health Organization (WHO) has reported that medical tourism "may facilitate access to high-level services by the better off; but it may also divert human resources from public services to more profitable private services for the elite or foreign markets, thus reducing staffing levels, lowering staff quality, and/or raising salary costs for the public sector." Private sector fees are also likely to rise correspondingly with the higher cost of medical tourism.

"Crowding in," on the other hand, suggests the possibility of medical tourism's benefits for public health through generalized economic gain and retention of doctors who might otherwise emigrate. Bookman and Bookman envision that "...a vibrant medical tourism industry can cooperate with the public sector so that non-paying patients can make use of facilities in the private sector. This might entail the cross-subsidization of one set of patients by another with respect to shared hospital beds, medical professionals' time and expertise, and diagnostic machinery." Only one such example is cited: "...in Chile where private insurance companies transfer member contributions to public health insurance to pay for indigent care." Hypothetically, profits from medical tourism could be allocated to strengthen public systems, but this Robin Hood scenario rests on an ethical imperative on the part of governments, corporations, and investors. As a third tier of ultra-privatized healthcare, medical tourism's influence on local access and quality of care has yet to be determined. Careful development of medical tourism, if regulated and taxed fairly, could provide revenues to ensure the sustainability and improvement of government health services. Alternatively, the danger exists for diversion of public resources to the more profitable practice of medicine for foreigners.

In Malaysia, the public sector still offers a high quality of care and choice of providers in a system that has proved remarkably effective in improving maternal health, child survival, and overall life expectancy. The key to these successes has been government commitment and financing, enabled by a strong and growing economy, and maintenance of a strong public system as a foundation for population health.

Low- and middle-income countries and transitional economies face critical choices in this time of deep crisis. Transnational healthcare offers a profitable avenue for bolstering threatened economies, but a recent Oxfam International report cites an important reminder that "No low- or middle-income country in Asia has achieved universal or near-universal access to healthcare without relying solely or predominantly on tax-funded public delivery." Medical tourism could be harnessed as a source of funding to strengthen public services, but only if decisive government action is joined with strong corporate responsibility.

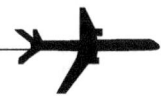

Regina Herzlinger
Professor
Harvard Business School

Regina Herzlinger
Professor
Harvard Business School

September 2009

Editor's Note: *The author of numerous books on healthcare, including* Who Killed Health Care?, Market-driven Health Care, *and* Consumer-driven Health Care, *Regina Herzlinger is one of the nation's most respected healthcare analysts. She is frequently called upon to contribute her opinions to numerous publications including* The Atlantic, Wall Street Journal, BusinessWeek, *and* The National Review.

She recently spoke with Medical Travel Today *regarding the future of the industry and its impact on both local and global economies.*

Medical Travel Today **(MTT): What will be the economic impact of medical tourism on the United States, as well as the global economy? Do you believe the projections for growth in medical travel are on target or "out of this world?"**

Regina Herzlinger (RH): I don't think the projections are too optimistic although it's hard to tell accurately what the exact number will be and it, of course, very much depends on what comes out of healthcare reform.

If we end up with a very centrally controlled healthcare reform, then medical tourism is unlikely to burgeon. This type of approach is simply unlikely to permit competition, which is so much what medical travel is about.

However, if we end up with universal coverage without a tightly controlled governmental infrastructure, clearly then there will be greater opportunity for medical travel. And this approach is doable: take a country like Switzerland that has universal coverage but no government program. It works wonderfully there. If we had this approach, it would lead to people finding the medical travel option attractive. The Swiss program allows for travel under their system and people do exercise the option.

However, if the care we get is government run, well, then the government makes the decisions, and those decisions would be more politically driven by special interest groups than true individual decisions. An individual will make a decision based on the value to them, whereas the government would be beholden to powerful stakeholders, including domestic hospitals, and, of course, unions. If the unions aren't in favor of global travel for care, it's unlikely to become an option for consumers.

All that said, I don't think we'll see a government-controlled program, but we will see expanded access. That is, consumers will have more options in terms of health insurance. Plus, there will be various tax remedies leading to more people buying health insurance for themselves.

MTT: Will government programs (Medicare/Medicaid) be likely to introduce medical travel options?

RH: No. They're typically laggards in adopting innovations because they are politically indebted to special interests that want to maintain the status quo and avoid the introduction of new competitors. They're very slow even when the benefits are obvious.

I think it will first advance through the private insurance sector. As it becomes clear that this is a do-good, do-well activity—that is, people get good care at good rates —then there will be pressure on the government to adopt it.

I think what we will eventually see is the Medicaid market going to places like Mexico and Costa Rica for care where there's a better value for their healthcare dollar, due to the fiscal pressure on the states that fund these programs and the large populations that are in the South.

The Medicare market, when it happens, is more likely to be worldwide, and not just Central and South America based.

MTT: Employer adoption of medical travel benefits has been slower than anticipated. Do you think that more employers will be looking to incorporate this type of benefit in 2009, 2010?

RH: The adoption curve for any innovation is typically 80/20. Upfront you've got companies like Hannaford, which is always an early mover on any healthcare service innovation. These types of companies are very innovative, an anomaly really, so in a way they don't count towards the statistics.

The way healthcare innovation adoption works is first you get 20 percent of employers on board. The next big group jumping on board accounts for another 20 percent, and then you get the laggards, the last 40 percent.

My gut is that the first 20 percent will be made up of large, self-insured companies that have trouble affording coverage. Large manufacturing companies have a terrific incentive to make it happen – but they're often unionized so it's not possible. But non-unionized employers, say construction and agriculture, they'll be the ones to make this happen. They have the economic incentive to do it.

You may see some medium or small companies, but their impact will be very small. Small companies are unlikely to do it unless medical travel facilitators become better at reaching out to them. For a CEO of a small company to arrange care abroad for her employees is simply too cumbersome.

Medium-sized companies, say less than 5,000 employees, would be good candidates for medical travel. They usually buy an insurance policy at a fixed price. In these situations if the insurance does not cover medical travel, no one's going to do it.

MTT: What are your thoughts on the idea that medical tourism negatively impacts local economies where the care is being provided? Do you perceive growth for the new breed of domestic medical travel?

RH: I can't get too excited about that. There's always the charge that you're catering to rich tourists. It's true for even resort hotels. But catering to the rich with medical travel allows local economies to learn a lot about how to bring quality care to the middle class citizens.

In India, for example, many hospital chains are geared toward the upper class and the medical tourist. As a result, they are organized very differently. Rather than an everything-for-everyone model, they have spokes for specialized facilities, hubs for high level care, and telemedicine. All this leads to a much more efficient delivery of healthcare, which ultimately brings more services to the middle and lower class.

Just look at the early history of the car industry. The first cars were built for the rich. At the time a car cost as much as a house. But pretty soon cars became largely middle class because of the efficiencies learned through the experience of building them for a few. The lessons learned by building for the upper class led to cars becoming accessible to the middle class.

I certainly think the argument is well intended, but it doesn't follow laws of economics. Most innovation is developed for specialized wealth sectors, but in the process you learn how to serve the middle class. You learn how to do whatever it is your doing— be it building cars or computers or delivering healthcare—very well, and as you drive down the cost, you become more efficient. That then makes it feasible to bring the service or product to the middle class and even the poor. They also have computers and cars.

In the short run, medical travel may displace services, but in the long run it will improve them.

The other thing to be mindful of is that when you cater and build to foreigners, this growth is largely being funded by external capital. That's not government money that's being spent there. And no matter how you look at that, it's good for the local economy.

It's essentially found money coming into their economy. Just look at India. Their entire gross domestic product is about a trillion dollars. The U.S. healthcare system alone is $2.3 trillion. How can they not gain from getting a piece of that?

MTT: What are the greatest opportunities for growth and development in the industry?
RH: Vendors might try targeting the mid-sized employers in the United States. I think that's an underpenetrated market. And as far as I know nobody is focusing on small employers. I understand that because it's very costly, but since most uninsured people would be prudently interested in healthcare savings, this would be a real opportunity area. Otherwise the industry, as far as the supply of facilities, is moving very well.

MTT: What countries/regions do you think are best poised to take advantage of these opportunities?
RH: That's an interesting question. I think countries have the opportunity to grow in the areas that are in synch with their local cultures. Cultures can really shape specialization.

Take Thailand for example. Thailand is the leading destination for gender alteration surgery, and that's largely because the Thais are so open and accepting of it. To them it's just correcting a natural mistake—a man born into a woman's body or vice versa. With that kind of culture, they are of course very good at that type of procedure and at understanding the patient needs.

Right now India is experiencing burgeoning prosperity and subsequently the diseases of prosperity. As it turns out, Indians also have a propensity for those diseases—diabetes and cardiovascular disease. It's really become an epidemic because as they've gotten more prosperous it's triggered what some might call a genetic proclivity. I think this makes India more likely to become the place to go for care in cardio and diabetes issues in the future. As in these examples, the centers of excellence in the future will reflect the cultural and medical needs of that culture.

MTT: What does the United States need to do to become a lead medical travel destination or to stop the outmigration of patients?

RH: You often hear people say that healthcare is local. There's no evidence of that. It's just a saying. We have no experience with what people really want to buy in healthcare because most of their expenses are shaped by insurers' choices.

We've seen that when people are motivated by economics, as per Hannaford, they're willing to send their employees to other states for care.

The U.S. market will also be driven by increased transparency. You know, I can sit here and read the label on my yogurt and tell you that it has 25 percent of the recommended calcium I need for the day, but I can't tell you who the best doctor in town is for a given procedure.

Pretty soon we'll have REAL transparency, like, how many people died when a doctor did a certain procedure, how many people got an infection at that hospital, how many medical errors were committed at that one. I'm talking about real data and outcomes. I recently needed toe surgery. I was told, "this guy's the best" and so on. Now, I value opinions, but when it comes right down to it I like to look at data. As it turns out I have a friend at a big insurer who sent me data about the doctors who do the type of surgery I needed on women my age. The doctor that was recommended to me had done zero. Zero! I ended up going to a different state to a different doctor who does 20 of these procedures a week. I didn't hesitate for one second to make that drive.

That kind of information should be available to everyone. People should be asking, "Why didn't I know the hospital had 40 percent infection rate?" It's a very valid question, and we should be furious that information is simply not out there.

In time we'll have greater transparency. The demand for it will be consumer-driven and the government will ultimately respond. It will be a huge driver for where people go for care.

The idea that healthcare is local is supported only by the absence of information.

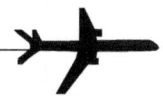

Paul Keckley
Executive Director
Deloitte Center for Health Solutions

January 2010

Editor's Note: *In 2008 the Deloitte Center for Health Solutions issued its first report on medical tourism. In October 2009, the Center issued an "update and implications" report that focused on the impact of the economy, the growth of foreign medical sites, the role of health plans to incentivize medical travel, and several other factors.*

Medical Travel Today *recently spoke with Paul Keckley, executive director, Deloitte Center for Health Solutions, to learn what the report revealed and how the industry needs to respond to both consumer and economic demands.*

Medical Travel Today **(MTT): What, if any, were the big surprises between your initial report and this most recent update?**
Paul Keckley (PK): I think there were two areas of particular surprise. First was the impact of the bad economy on the industry. We found a substantial slow down in the number of elective procedures.

In our survey of consumers, we found one out of five saying that even though they have need for gum surgery or a carpal tunnel surgery, they're choosing to delay tending to it. That choice is a direct result of the economy.

Second, we were surprised to find that employer groups were not aggressively promoting medical tourism. There are companies out there that are introducing medical tourism options in their benefits, but it's not an across-the-board component in the arsenal of offerings for most companies.

This hesitation can actually be tied back to the economy, too. If you're an employer and in the last 24 months you've been cutting benefits and having to lay-off staff, well, then you're spending more time thinking about survival and competition than you are about substantially changing your benefits. But let me add that there was a bright spot in the study and that had to do with the maturity of the industry. We saw this as a very strong positive.

When we first looked at the industry in 2006, we found that there wasn't much clinically coordinated care. That is, there wasn't much pre- and post-operative reporting, outcomes reporting, and capturing of data. Now, were finding the industry maturing around clinical processes. We refer to this new approach as Medical Tourism 2.0.

That's not to say that everybody in the industry is doing it well. In fact, the rank and file medical tourism operator is nowhere near the level of transparency that they need to be. But among the more established programs, they are definitely getting there, and it is beginning to truly separate them from the rest.

It's clear to us that there is a movement to make more data available and in the end, that will be a boost to the industry

MTT: The lack of a governing body for international care continues to surface as an issue that could inhibit growth. What group or organization do you see in the best position to fill this gap, or do you think a new body needs to be formed?

PK: I've gone to meetings of various groups and it appears that the Medical Travel Association (MTA) is maybe in the best position -- but I think it's still early.

The challenge there is that a trade association that focuses on professional development shouldn't cross lines into being a commercial association that sells service and does a lot of other things.

It should be either a standard setting organization that advances the professional integrity of the business or a trade group that develops a set of goods or services it sells. I think the MTA needs to figure out what they want to be.

But I don't see any other group quite as far along or as close to potentially being a standard setting group. Whether or not the MTA chooses to go that route or the commercial route remains to be seen.

MTT: You cited inbound medical travel as the subset slated for the slowest growth. Given the health care reform measures, do you think trying to stimulate inbound growth is a realistic or even a good idea?

PK: I don't think that any increase in inbound travel would be a result of medical reform. It's more likely an increase would be the result of better marketing and a high value proposition. At this point marketing has to be highly targeted.

The growth of the market will be primarily in the commercial market where people have a high-deductible insurance product.

The outbound medical travel market will increasingly focus on potential cost savings for low-risk ambulatory surgical procedures and becoming attractive to young adults with commercial insurance.

MTT: I found it interesting that the two states that had bills to incentivize medical tourism were landlocked states. Does geography really have anything to do with driving the desire for a bill or is it more of a reflection on the level of care available in a state?

PK: The latter. The current bent of consumers considering medical tourism is directly linked first to proximity and second to direct air coverage. Those residing in states that border Mexico will naturally consider Mexico. Those seeking a procedure on the eastern seaboard, especially those in Florida, Georgia, and South Carolina, will make their decisions based on the availability of direct flights to the Caribbean. Medical tourism also maps to people's use of the internet for self-care and willingness to use retail clinics as a substitute for primary care.

MTT: Are there any countries you consider to be "ones to watch"?

PK: I think the two most intriguing efforts are being made in South Korea and potentially Dubai and the United Arab Emirates (UAE).

Europeans view Dubai and the UAE as a very close and desirable option. South Korea has attracted a global following of expats who are working or living somewhere else and willing to come back for care.

The advantage these two locations have over the established ones is that they are starting with the Medical Travel 2.0 model. They're using technology to coordinate referrals and aftercare, and they're capturing data.

From a strategic marketing standpoint, they're targeting employers and health plans rather than individual consumers. In other words, they're swinging a bigger bat.

Plus, they're specializing. They are looking at particular patient population and focusing on it. They're building their expertise and building high-volume, low-price options that appeal to consumers.

Another area to keep an eye on is dental. Up until now it has largely flown under the radar. But as dental benefits get dropped, consumers are being completely surprised by the cost for surgical procedures in dentistry. I see this as a huge growth market that's currently untapped in medical tourism.

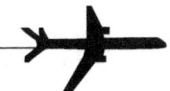

Brian Boxer Wachler, M.D.
Ophthalmologist
Boxer Wachler Vision Institute

May 2010

Editor's Note: *Medical travel professionals watching the Vancouver Winter Olympic games had an extra reason to cheer this year. In addition to witnessing the power of training and commitment by world-class athletes, those who watched the men's bobsled also witnessed the power of medical travel.*

In 2007, Steve Holcomb, driver of the U.S. mens' four-man bobsled, was going blind due to a degenerative eye condition called Keratoconus. He was told the only hope of regaining his vision was a corneal transplant. While offering promising results, a transplant was invasive and the results would be fragile in nature, meaning it would not help Holcomb regain the ability to drive again. However, the U.S. Bobsled Federation wasn't ready to give up its best driver just yet. Instead, they researched and discovered a new, non-surgical procedure called C3-R treatment.

As described by Brian Boxer Wachler, M.D., who pioneered the treatment, C3-R "uses vitamin applications and light to strengthen the cornea...and cure the disease without the need for a cornea transplant." The treatment takes 30 minutes and is performed in a doctor's office without anesthesia.

In December 2007, Holcomb traveled 700 miles to the Boxer Wachler Vision Institute to undergo the treatment. The results were nothing short of miraculous for Steve and the team. Thanks to the treatment and a pair of implantable contact lenses used to further enhance Holcomb's vision, Holcomb not only resumed his driver position on the U.S. four-man bobsled team, he steered the team to gold – the first U.S. bobsled medal of any color in 50 years.

Medical Travel Today *spoke with Dr. Boxer Wachler about the C3-R treatment and his role in this great Olympic story.*

***Medical Travel Today* (MTT): First, congratulations on your contribution towards helping the United States Bobsled team bring home its first medal, and a gold one at that, in 50 years.**
Dr. Brian Boxer Wachler (BBW): Thank you. I can't express to you what an absolute thrill it was to be there and witness Steve and his team cross that finish line. I really did cry like a baby when we knew they had taken the gold. And honestly, I was just one of many people who helped the dream come true.

MTT: Yes, I understand that it was the bobsled team and Olympic committee that really made the dream possible.
BBW: That's right. Steve had actually retired from the sport for two years because of the issue with his eyes.

Meanwhile the U.S. Olympic committee was trying to get the team ready for Vancouver. They asked, "what do you need to win?" Steve's teammates basically said, "We need Steve." They recognized that he was the best driver ever in the history of the

U.S. team. They told the Olympic committee that their best chance at gold was with Steve. The committee then turned around and charged the team doctor, Dr. Stoll, with finding a way to get Steve in driving form.

When Steve was first diagnosed, it was recommended he get a corneal transplant. The procedure can certainly be very effective, but it would not allow him to ever drive a sled again. That wasn't going to work.

Dr. Stoll began looking for alternatives and found me. I looked at Steve's records and then examined him and determined he was a good candidate for the C3-R procedure. In reality, he got that procedure paired with a vitamin application and light treatment. Then three months later he received implantable contacts in both eyes just to further refine his vision.

MTT: We learned through the media that Steve Holcomb's procedure was not covered by insurance. Is that true for all patients seeking this procedure?
BBW: C3-R is typically an out-of-pocket expense. But even so, I perform it on a weekly basis and pretty much have for the past six years.

When it comes to sight, people are quite willing to pay what they can and travel as far as they need to retain or regain it.

MTT: From where do your patients come and how do they find you?
BBW: They literally come from all over the world. Most find me by simply doing research on the web. I do enough papers and presentations on the topic that my name tends to pop up.

I've also authored a book, Modern Management of Keratoconus and the Lasik Consumer Report. Once they get my name, they can find my websites (Boxerwachler. com, www.KeratoconusInserts.com).

MTT: Do most of your patients work through a facilitator?
BBW: No, my office handles many of the arrangements for them. We started treating international patients about seven years ago…even before C3-R. At that time we simply began making arrangements for their travel, lodging, sightseeing, and so on. Now we have a fairly comprehensive system in place.

MTT: Do you currently work with medical travel facilitators?
BBW: Not presently, but I'd be happy to consider working with them. My focus is on performing procedure to save or regain sight, not facilitating travel. If I can find partners who want to help bring more patients in for procedures, I'm all for it.

MTT: What kind of services do you offer pre- or post-care, specifically for patients travelling great distances?
BBW: We'll see them for a minimum of three days. Generally one day in advance of the procedure to do a final exam and handle pre-op procedures. Then one day for the procedure and one-day of post-op. That's the absolute minimum. My staff will also arrange for follow-up care at home.

That sounds short, but I've typically had a lot of contact before they arrive, reviewing records and imaging. Before they board the plane we've established a preliminary recommendation.

MTT: So with C3-R only one procedure is necessary?
BBW: In 99 percent of the cases, only one treatment is needed.

MTT: What is the typical out-of-pocket expense for C3-R?
BBW: We do offer patients financing options through different companies. This way they're in for a few hundred dollars per month versus the whole nut up front. It's something that many, many patients appreciate and access. Of course each case is different but typically it's about $3,100 per eye.

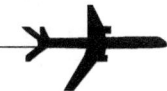

Armando Baez
President
Global Benefits Group, International Claim Services

May 2010

Editor's Note: *Armando Baez is president of the International Claim Services division of Global Benefits Group, the world's largest independent, fully integrated provider of international benefits, and acts as general manager of GBG's China subsidiary. He is also chairman of the Board of the Self-Insurance Institute of America, Inc. (SIIA). These roles provide him with a unique perspective on the medical travel industry.* Medical Travel Today *recently spoke with him to get his take on the industry's evolution and how employers are responding.*

***Medical Travel Today* (MTT): If you would, please briefly tell us about Global Benefits Group and SIIA and how they intersect with medical travel.**
Armando Baez (AB): Global Benefits Group is a specialty insurer offering health, disability, and life coverage for people working outside their home countries. For these folks, medical travel is simply their normal benefit and what we've helped them do for the past 30 years. We developed a World Medical Network through which our clients get care. We've refined our list of providers pretty tightly so we know that our clients are getting the best care in every corner of the globe. I guess in some sense, we're probably the most established organization in medical travel around.

SIIA, on the other hand, is new to the international stage even though SIIA is the leading association for employers engaged in self-insurance or alternative-risk transfer insurance. The rising cost of traditional health care and workers' compensation insurance has driven more employers to look at self-insured options because of the savings they can realize and the greater control over their unique risks. In the past few years, medical travel, or what we prefer to call "Global Medical" has become another cost-saving benefit that's being given more and more consideration by this self-insured group of buyers.

MTT: Given that you have a seasoned understanding of medical travel based on your Global Benefits experience, I'm curious what observations or questions you might have about how medical travel continues to evolve for the 'rest of the world'?
AB: The one thing I've been surprised is that the medical tourism industry has become more like the travel agency industry than a preferred provider network. So often you hear "we can arrange for your travel from here to there" rather than taking a "we have a global network of care to offer" approach.

In my opinion, the right approach to take this industry to the next level is a global preferred provider one, and not the boutique tourist agency one.

You know, PPO networks in the U.S. are already engaged in the preferred provider approach. They just tend to have a very regional or localized view. There's no reason a PPO can't have a network that spans a continent, a hemisphere, or even the globe. They can leave it up to consumers to decide how far they want to go, the same way they currently choose to go in- or out-of-network. We should present the associated cost, the advantages of care, and so on and then let the member decide… it's really the same thing they're currently doing but with bigger boundaries. Or, in one sense, no boundaries…that's why SIIA prefers to call this movement "Global Health" and not Medical Tourism.

MTT: What kind of attention is SIIA paying to medical travel at this point?
AB: SIIA launched an international committee to take self-insurance education and promotion global. At every conference we hold, "Global Health" is a big, big topic. This year we'll be hosting our 30th Annual National Educational Conference & Expo in Chicago. The "Global Health" topic will be addressed in both the international and health care education tracks. I would expect those presentations to be very well attended.

Everyone wants to understand how "Global Health" works—what it is, what its benefits and risks are, and so on. I would also expect that, given the reach SIIA has in the self insurance industry globally, we'll be seeing an increase in the number of medical travel companies represented in the exhibitor space. I hope to engage them in a dialogue about the direction of this industry and what we can do to solve its inherent problems, which are preventing buyers from signing up in bigger numbers.

MTT: What do you think are the ongoing concerns and objections of SIIA members to medical travel? How have they changed in the past few years?
AB: At a high level, there are two things the industry needs to overcome. The first is the name "medical tourism." It simply conveys the wrong message. You're not a tourist. You're an individual with a medical issue looking for care. I think vendors do a disservice to the industry when they bill themselves as a medical tourism operator. This is why I prefer to call it "Global Health."

The second is that the industry is built on a concept that "I'll save you a lot of money, and I'll make money off the savings." Consumers and benefit plan sponsors aren't stupid. This kind of financing model creates a liability for our industry. If, as a medical travel operator, I'm going to incentivize you to go somewhere cheaper for care in order for me to make more money from the difference, the consumer has to question where quality comes into the equation. This kind of I win-you lose model sets the consumer up for a bad experience. No industry can afford bad consumer experiences at any level.

MTT: I understand the SIIA is having a meeting in London. Are you expanding your reach to be global?
AB: SIIA just concluded a successful meeting in Singapore exploring alternative risk transfer solutions for companies doing business in South and East Asia. Before that we met in Barcelona and also toured China. Essentially, we're trying to take self insurance and alternative risk transfer concepts into the international arena to teach others how to do self-insurance right. We want people to understand how self-insurance can be a part of their risk management initiatives.

It is becoming clear that a lot of countries around the world have relied on government run insurance schemes, and they're not working. For example, China is doing everything it can to promote private health care and already allows for self-insurance. It has to be said that government-run insurance does not work. It works as a redistribution of wealth mechanism—just look at England and Canada—but, for lack of a better phrase, it dumbs down the level of health care. When everybody gets the same, some get what they didn't have before, but most get less than they used to have. I predict that is what is about to happen in the U.S.

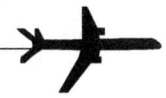

Paula Wilson
President & Chief Executive Officer

Paul van Ostenberg
Executive Director
Joint Commission International

July 2010

Editor's Note: *There's a new and highly articulate president at the Joint Commission International — a champion for health care quality and continuous improvement at every junction of the delivery system.*

In an exclusive interview with Paula Wilson, Medical Travel Today *publisher and executive editor Laura Carabello gets a sneak preview of what's in store for JCI and what lies ahead for international accreditation.*

Additional comments from Paul van Ostenberg, executive director, Department of Standards Development and Interpretation at JCI, provide a better understanding of the organization's intensity regarding standards.

The following is Part One of the interview.

Medical Travel Today **(MTT): Congratulations, Paula, on your new leadership role with JCI. I'd like to get a sense from you, is it going to be business as usual, or do you see changes at JCI?**
Paula Wilson (PW): It's an interesting question because when you say, "Is it business as usual?" – JCI's core business is focused on patient safety and quality health care, so that doesn't change at all. That's obviously the mission of the organization and continues to be our central focus in terms of how we're running what is already a very good organization. I certainly would like to think I am going to bring some strengths and some new ideas and visions that are going to take a really, really, good organization to the next level. We're constantly looking for ways to do better, and I see that as part of my responsibilities, as well. In terms of what we do, our business of accreditation, consulting, and education complement other activities. We are going to stay the course in terms of those activities.

MTT: When you say you're going to bring new ideas and visions to the organization, what specifically do you have in mind?
PW: That's still a work in progress, some of which is looking at all the ways to make the organization more efficient and running well from an operational perspective. From a different perspective, there are other ways to do what were are doing in terms of: What is the current focus in terms of our business model? What are we doing well and that we can do more of? What could we do better? I'm still relatively new on the job and am exploring the possibilities.

MTT: What are your perspectives on the growth of the industry?

PW: There seems to be a trend of growth, but I would not cite numbers because there isn't a specific way of tracking patients. There is certainly a trend that exists today which did not exist ten years ago. From a Joint Commission or Joint Commission International perspective, this is a neutral issue. It's not something that we are in the business to track or be a part of, but it has driven certain organizations around the world to come to us seeking accreditation. Because of our mission and dedication to patient safety, we accommodate those requests and accredit hospitals involved in medical tourism.

An intriguing question often asked is, "Do you think that health reform in the U.S. is a positive, neutral, or negative factor for medical tourism around the world?" If you go with the theory that some people are medical tourists because of cost issues in the United States -- which may, in fact, be the case – this is likely to change after the full implementation of health reforms.

MTT: You're not prepared to even make that prognostication?
PW: I think it's an intellectual, interesting, and relevant issue, but I can't even begin to speculate. We don't know enough about the actual implementation of the health reform package and the impact it will have. We keep talking about medical tourism as a United States phenomenon, but there are medical tourists all over the world and the U.S. health reforms have no impact on the decisions to seek cross-border care in other countries. Since there are people who come to the U.S. for care, and there are people within Europe who go to other European countries for care, this is not purely a domestic issue.

MTT: Well, except that everyone looks at the U.S. as the golden goose. They all want the U.S. market but don't know how to access it. I hear it all the time from countries that say they would like to get the U.S. patient.
PW: I'm not surprised at that: it makes sense on some level.

MTT: They believe that the numbers are there and the timing right, especially with U.S. health care reform. It's interesting that you say it's not time yet to make that determination.
PW: If health reform is implemented perfectly, and health care costs in the U.S. go down for the patient or the consumer, would that then make it less imperative to look outside of the country to get care? I don't know.

MTT: What people are saying is that health care reform is not going to drive down health care costs.
PW: I think that people who have been very involved in writing and passing the law are optimistic about the cost curve. We'll see what happens.

MTT: I hear all the time about the cost of JCI accreditation and that all the other accreditation programs are less expensive. Why should hospitals spend money to get accredited or reaccredited by JCI?
PW: First of all, I think there is some misinformation about cost. When you do an apples-to-apples comparison, we're pretty price-competitive, especially if you're going to compare the cost of the JCI survey to another organization that uses paid surveyors. When the accreditation organization uses a group of volunteer surveyors, there is no question that there's going to be a price differential because they're not paying

the surveyors. I would argue that the quality of the survey is different in that instance -- and I'll leave it at that.

The other point is that surveys cost money because sometimes we uncover things that require improvement. For instance, we help the organization to understand that perhaps they need new equipment, which can in turn drive new expenditures. These are residual costs that come from a survey because of our findings, and improvement of health care is the result of an investment made by the hospital.

Another point that never gets discussed in this context is the fact that over time, delivering safe, high quality patient care gets a really good return on investment. It's certainly a positive not only for the patient, but also for the providers, as well and the hospitals. These expenditures need to be viewed as an investment in their future -- in terms of not only doing more business but also improving the way they provide care and saving money over the long haul.

If you look at JCI in comparison to others, look at the bigger picture. The cost of the survey is one line item, but it will pay tremendous dividends when you factor in the return on investment.

MTT: Do you have an economic model?
PW: We've done some work on the value of accreditation from an economic perspective, but we're not finished with that research yet. We just completed the first pilot study in Lebanon and started the second pilot study in Thailand.
Paul van Ostenberg (PVO): There appears to be some confusion in the field of accreditation. The International Society for Quality in Healthcare accredits the accrediting bodies, and people presume that if we're all accredited by ISQUA, we're the same. This is not the case. It means that we meet a set of similar principals, but if we go much deeper than that, we have different ways that we develop standards. For example, JCI's standards are developed with a panel of experts from every continent around the globe.

Our on-site methodology is different, and we set the bar at different heights. We use different techniques for evaluating the level of compliance with standards, and we have different decision rules. I would argue that we are very different from all the other accrediting bodies. For example, we don't use a self-assessment. Others rely primarily on a self-assessment by the organization with some on-site validation, while we are inside the health care organization conducting rigorous evaluations by trained surveyors. Ours is a very different model.

We have spent a few years developing standards with an international task force. JCI's standards are unique and designed specifically for the international market, whereas other accreditors try to use their own national standards and apply them internationally. We also generate better standards through regional advisory councils, and we have a whole different structure of getting input into the standards themselves. While other organizations may seem to have a quicker and easier route to accreditation, it is because they employ a very different methodology. We believe that if JCI accreditation is going to be achieved by a specific organization, we have to be with them on the front lines of patient care. We have to interview caregivers, administrators, and patients... we have to examine key documents... we have to observe care... we have to conduct intensive on-site examination of the processes. We believe that our approach goes way beyond a self-assessment process.

MTT: Would you care to mention any of the other accreditation bodies by name? Are there others that you feel are similar to or different from JCI?

PW: I know all of them because we sit together on the accreditation council of ISQUA. Every accreditation body is unique and unto itself. We see different accrediting bodies in different parts of the world, and each one chooses the parts of the world where they would like to work. We encounter our accreditation colleagues all over the globe.

MTT: So you feel that there isn't one other that's the same caliber as JCI?
PW: We're comfortable saying that JCI is the leading accreditor for patient care and patient safety. In fact, the other accrediting bodies come to us to learn. For example, we've taught the patient tracer methodology to several other accrediting bodies throughout the world. We used it for two to three years before others came to us to learn.

MTT: Tell me a little about the patient tracer.
PVO: It really evaluates an organization on the way that they care for patients by tracing a particular patient. We evaluate the ways in which the health care organization coordinates care, makes care decisions, plans care, and implements care. We trace different types of patients, tracking them from the emergency room through surgery. We interview everybody who has touched the patient and made a decision.

It's important to look at the communications among caregivers and all documentation of essential patient information. JCI really established this methodology, including system tracers that "trace" the medication management system. We actually trace high-risk medications throughout the organization, how they are used, policies regarding their utilization, and the level of staff understanding about their use. We trace information as it weaves its way through the organization. We use tracers in more ways than other accrediting bodies -- we have taught others about patient tracers, and we've made innovations ever since.

MTT: I don't think a lot of the market is aware of this.
PW: JCI strives to be as transparent as possible and put valuable information on our Website (www.jointcommissioninternational.org) where it's available for the public to review. We share this type of information when we attend the ISQUA meetings.

MTT: From the employer and payer perspectives, is their confidence in JCI justified?
PVO: JCI seeks to continually set the mark for patient safety higher and higher. We do that with our standards and our decision rules, and we're creating performance measures. Several hospitals have successfully gone through the JCI accreditation process three times, and they are asking, "What's next?"

We are working on 'what's next' and that's an important part of our progress over the next few years – to continually set the pace for accrediting bodies. All the hospitals and health care organizations we work with learn from each other, and we've developed a group of loyal customers. In fact, our retention rate is 98 percent. The reason a health care organization drops out of JCI accreditation is primarily because they have been sold or merged. We have a high retention rate because we work to provide the greatest value to the organization going through the process.

MTT: You don't get a lot of pushback on the price?
PVO: No. What we do get are questions about the variable costs -- that's the travel involved with getting a team of surveyors into a country. We've taken some steps to

modify this amount: We now have trained surveyors living around the world who can survey in neighboring countries. As a result, our travel costs per survey are steadily decreasing. We also cluster surveys, meaning that when we go into a country we can conduct three or four surveys allowing the organizations to split the travel expenses.

We are making every effort to reduce the variable costs. If you take five people and send them for five days into a hospital, you'll probably incur the same costs across all accrediting bodies. Actually, if you look at International Organization for Standardization (ISO), it's sometimes even more expensive to take that route to accreditation. So, we're working very hard to keep the variable costs down.

MTT: I think people need to understand that too. Let's spend a little time now on accreditation for outpatient facilities. Do you think this is of growing importance?
PW: Absolutely. The phenomenon of moving patients to outpatient settings is worldwide. More and more sophisticated procedures are being performed on an outpatient basis, and we have just revised all of our ambulatory standards (available here: http://www.jointcommissioninternational.org/Accreditation-Manuals/JCI-ACCREDITA-TION-STANDARDS-FOR-PRIMARY-CARE/476/). We've also developed a set of primary care standards. Some countries don't really have an ambulatory system, but they have a primary care system.

Between the primary care and the ambulatory care settings, many big health care systems are seeking JCI accreditation. In Spain, for example, it might be a whole region that will seek for accreditation of the 50 or so primary care providers in the region. We do have a new program that can accredit these networks. All of these standards are available on the JCI Web site with most of the detail.

Editor's Note: *The following is Part Two of an exclusive interview with Paula Wilson and Paul van Ostenberg of Joint Commissions International conducted by Laura Carabello, publisher of* Medical Travel Today.

Medical Travel Today (MTT): Let's spend a little time now on accreditation for outpatient facilities. Do you think this is of growing importance?
Paula Wilson (PW): Absolutely. The phenomenon of moving patients to outpatient settings is worldwide. More and more sophisticated procedures are being performed on an outpatient basis, and we have just revised all of our ambulatory standards.

We've also developed a set of primary care standards. Some countries don't really have an ambulatory system, but they have a primary care system. Between the primary care and the ambulatory care settings; many big health care systems are seeking JCI accreditation. In Spain, for example, it might be a whole region that will seek for accreditation of the 50 or so primary care providers in the region. We do have a new program that can accredit these networks. All of these standards are available on the JCI Web site with most of the detail.

Paul van Ostenberg (PVO): JCI has gone above and beyond by publishing standards since the very beginning, making them available on the Web site in the public domain. What's happened is that a lot of national accrediting bodies have developed standards similar to ours, and that's okay. That reflects JCI's mission to continuously improve the safety and quality of care in the international community.

MTT: So there's a lot of look-a-likes out there?
PVO: Just because other accrediting bodies have similar standards doesn't mean they

are exactly like us. All of our algorithms for making accreditation decisions based on those standards can be quite different. You can take the same the set of standards and set the bar really low -- and it can be easy to become accredited. We set the bar quite high, and about one quarter of the organizations that are surveyed for the first time do not meet the decision rules for achieving accreditation. When this happens, our surveyors to go back within 90 days and gather more information to see if the improvement they made now meets JCI's requirements.

MTT: Could outpatient surgical centers owned by physicians get together and apply for accreditation as a group?
PW: Actually, under certain conditions they could. What we mean by a network is that there is a central office, and that all of the different clinical care sites are under the same management, follow the same policies and the same protocols -- more like a franchise. It's a governance issue.

MTT: So it wouldn't be 10 plastic surgeons in Rio de Janeiro that got together said, "Let's get accredited."
PW: You're right...that's not it. There may be primary care clinics that are distributed throughout a country, as is the case in Saudi Arabia where ambulatory clinics are all over. What's different here is that you can survey certain functions performed by a central office -- governance, leadership, policy development and deployment communication monitoring the quality of care across the network. Then JCI surveys a sampling of the actual provider sites, and selects the sample based upon location, differences in population, and differences in services. While much of the operation is highly centralized, we need to visit a sampling of the provider sites.

MTT: How many facilities do you envision will become accredited or re-accredited in the next one, two or five years' time?
PW: We now have about 345 accredited hospitals, and they are on the three-year cycle. With that number, we expect about 100 to come back for their triennial survey next year. So with approximately 100 hospitals per year seeking re-accreditation, and annual growth of about 25-30 percent, there appears to be a continuing growth trend. When we introduce a new program there's an uptick. Today, there is a lot of the growth in primary care accreditation. There is also growth within certain countries.

MTT: Is the majority of your business coming from a particular part of the world? For example is India more active with accreditation then let's say Japan?
PW: There's no real trend for this, but that's one of the interesting things I am excited to learn more about – identifying geographic trends or in certain provider types. We're learning about these trends as we go along.

JCI can influence a trend by how we translate our standards. Currently, we have 15 different languages for hospital accreditation, and we recently translated into Japanese. We've accredited the leading hospital in Japan, and we're hiring Japanese-speaking surveyors. As a result of the standards translation, we expect that the Japanese market is going to boom for us in the next few years, and we've invested in more Japanese-centric capabilities.

All the languages are available on our Web site. Korean is the latest language to be added and we plan to translate the site into many more languages.

MTT: Have you tackled Portuguese?

PVO: Yes, and we have two Portuguese translations—Brazilian and Portuguese. It's interesting that there are two versions. The people in Portugal people believe that the Brazilians speak a modern kind of Portuguese.

MTT: Do you see a growth of activity in Central-South and Latin America -- or even the Caribbean Islands?

PVO: We do. We have been getting a lot more requests and interest in Mexico, Chile and Peru, and it is spreading. We do not have an office in Central or South America, but we do have an accreditation partner in Brazil.

MTT: Who is that?

PVO: Associação Brasileira de Acreditação de Sistemas e Serviços de Saúde (ABA), previously known as the Consortium for Brazilian Accreditation (CBA), is our accreditation partner in Brazil. ABA is a duplicate of the JCI central office in Chicago. They have the same standards and rules, and we share an accreditation committee. They put on all the educational conferences, and we survey the organizations together. They really have been our face for Brazil, which is an enormous country.

MTT: Are you going to be speaking at any upcoming international meetings?

PW: We're still working on our schedules, but are not sure of the specifics of where and when. That's starting to all come together.

PVO: There is a group of meetings that we help to sponsor, such as Health Management Asia – this year in South Korea, for which we are a corporate sponsor. We participate very heavily in the ISQUA meeting and at its annual meeting coming up in Paris during October.

PW: We also put on our own series of meetings in October: Executive briefings in three locations -- Barcelona, Singapore and Dubai. These are designed to update standards for all accreditation organizations worldwide. We heavily support the continuing flow of education on standards, accreditation policies and information on compliance. It keeps our business growing.

MTT: Is the JCI gold standard in the international marketplace expected to continue?

PW: Absolutely. I think everything we have said points in that direction, particularly around the standards themselves. We have international standards, and if you look at what we do and the value we bring to organizations, the demand for our survey and our accreditation will surely build as we continue to get better. That's our goal-- to only be better than we already are.

PVO: JCI accreditation leaves a bigger impact on patient quality and safety. It also means bringing more value to the organization for going through the process. That's something we are asking ourselves all the time in terms of customer service and in terms of making sure we are responding to the right demands of hospitals and other providers. We are extremely relevant to their business and to the safety of their patients. To this point, we have launched a portal on our Web site where anybody can ask a question regarding the standards, and it's monitored 24-7. Standard compliance questions are answered very quickly in a format that is easily used for implementation.

MTT: Do you see US employers and payers finally opting for medical travel benefits and will JCI accreditations help them move forward?

PW: Our mission is not related to medical tourism, or how US companies provide health care for their employees. Those are the external trends that are happening; while they are relevant to us, they are not what we spend our time thinking about.

We do spend our time thinking about patients, quality and safety. So if the trend continues, we are prepared to become responsive to providers and to help them be prepared for that trend. I don't think anyone knows what US employers will do. It's interesting, because you don't mention the patients themselves. They're part of that decision-making process, as well. I don't think there is enough data to judge how big this trend will become. I know employers have a great deal of concern over how employees access health care. This is new territory and I don't know how they're making those decisions: Which employees are opting to travel, which procedures they would consider and what locations are most attractive. For us, medical travel is something that's happening, and it means that there is a need for us to respond to provider requests.

PVO: When we accredit a hospital, we don't pay attention to where the patient comes from. We presume that a patient who lives in the shadow of the hospital gets the same high quality care as the patient who travels from another country. So we really look at the entire patient population. We do not sample all patient records or anything based upon whether the patient is from another country -- it just doesn't enter into our methodology at all. But we are doing things that are helping organizations to justify the quality of their care. For example, we now have a cardiac surgery benchmark indicator project and are testing the Internet-based software. Currently, we're in 15 hospitals in 6 different countries collecting cardiac surgery outcomes. Based upon this, we'll be able to start looking at orthopedic outcomes, cancer outcomes and other areas.

We expect to develop broader capabilities that help organizations to benchmark their care -- and that's the kind of information that will be a part of the decision-making process for purchasers in the future. But it's also a core process that we want these organizations to engage in for their own improvement. If they can use that kind of information for other benefits, it's fine; but we're concerned that they learn from it and keep improving their performance (i.e., cardiac surgery) based upon having good outcomes data.

MTT: If you had to give hospitals a couple of pieces of advice regarding how to prepare for JCI accreditation, what would you say?

PW: I would start with a visit to our Web site, which is a very good resource and very informative. Start looking at our publications – there is a newer one that explains how to prepare for JCI accreditation. We make these very user- friendly and highly accessible. They should do some homework and research, and look at what we're making available on the Web.

PVO: We also conduct a series of programs around the world called Practicum. They are one- week, intensive experiences that include going to see a box survey in a hospital. So, if they are curious about all of the content around the standards, as well as the whole process, they can attend a Practicum. We are doing about six or eight of these annually around the world.

MTT: Anything that I didn't ask that you think our market place should know?

PW: I think that the culture of the Joint Commission and Joint Commission International is using evidence to improve care, that's a core value of our entire enterprise. I think organizations that are interested in us, learning from us and are participating with us on any level are, hopefully, embracing this value, as well.

PVO: We are trying to -- and are making a specific effort right now -- to really drive evidence in the design of the standards. We're looking at patient outcomes, and the purpose of these accreditations is to make the patient outcomes positive. I think that organizations that embrace that kind of culture and that kind of value can be aligned with us. I would certainly emphasize that message. We're continually trying to understand what makes high performance organizations do so well, and pull this information so that we can teach others.

We are an education and learning organization. It is evident that health care won't be the same in five years, and we will be ahead of that curve. We will be at the top of the discussion, in terms of being relevant to health care organizations and in terms of the current practice and issues in health care.

MTT: I think one of the trends we are seeing is that reimbursement and payment will be tied to performance-based outcomes.

PW: Exactly -- that is something our enterprise is thinking about.

MTT: We haven't even talked about US domestic medical, and promoting these opportunities. What is your viewpoint?

PVO: As much as we can help to base it on good data, we will. JCI has a brand new standard -- if any of our accredited organizations posts clinical outcome data on its Web site, the data must be validated and the leaders of the organization are responsible to insure that they only publish valid data. There has been no monitoring of that -- and some of the data I see is very suspect.

MTT: Who should be validating that data?

PVO: We think that should be a capability that is inside any good organization. You collect data, you validate it, and you analyze it, and make decisions on it. But organizations aren't very good at that, so we have new standards to build that capacity to validate their data when it's appropriate. For example, when something seems to be changing or you're putting in a new clinical measure, you need to make sure that you are collecting it correctly and that it's valid. There are third parties that can validate the data, too. But we want to be able to build this capability so that it becomes an internal capacity, as part of quality improvement -- not something you buy from an external source.

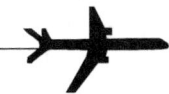

Fred Hunt
President
Society of Professional Benefit Administrators

September 2010

Medical Travel Today **(MTT): Give me a thumbnail about your organization and its growth.**
Fred Hunt (FH): There are third party administrators and firms that are hired by client employee benefit plans and employers of every size and format, which puts us in a unique situation. I feel funny saying this, but while we're a small operation, we are the largest — meaning that about 52 to 55 percent of U.S. workers with coverage are with plans administered by our members.

What is unique is that TPAs are in an advisory position with every kind of self-funded plan, including union, non-union, big and small employers, government entities, and even some native tribes and some new things such as prison systems. We have received a few calls from the local hospitals, and they call TPAs and say, "Hey, it's not a plan obviously, but can you help us manage the medical costs and all?" The role that we play is that we try to stay under the radar in terms of remaining non-political, non- partisan. We are a type of resource for the government, and we have a very close relationship. They will often call upon us and say, "Here is the direction we are thinking about going in…what would happen if…" What would work for a single employer plan might work for a government plan. That's what we do.

As far as the future of TPAs, I think our demise has been predicted every year for the past 30 years. I have been here and it hasn't happened. The reason is that we're in the red tape business, and as long as there is red tape — and we know that there will always be red tape -- our business will flourish. Also, the real key to the TPA business is personalization, and that kicks in on the travel issue, as well. People often approach me with ideas that make absolutely perfect business sense, and yet they flop. The reason is that human nature issues -- not business concerns – come into play. But, because our members are very sensitive to their plans and their needs, and our clients are very attentive to what their workers want, we sometimes end up being the messenger of bad news.

I often describe our office as the fire department. It will often seem slow and then all of a sudden all hell breaks loose. We get about 2,000 or more calls from members and people a year, a month, and every week.

MTT: What is your knowledge of the medical travel market place, and how do you see it positioned in 2010 and beyond?
FH: I see medical travel as one of several different kinds of things — old and new — which are available and make perfect, logical sense. But then they have to face the challenge of the human nature test. I'm often reminded of centers of excellence. About 20 years ago, you could go to the center of excellence for the best service in the country for less money, and employers were willing to pay for you to go. I remember doing this for a group of businesses, and there was this elderly senior woman who said,

" I can't leave my grandbabies!" This became the problem: People would say, "No! No! I'm going to a county hospital rather than the best clinic because I don't want to be far from people in the family."

I repeated this to some of my organization members, and they said they had the same anecdotes. One woman had remarked, "My husband wouldn't know what to do if he couldn't come to ask me where the things in the kitchen were located." As a result, the centers of excellence thing kind of fizzled. Being a long-term skeptic, that is my concern. What really makes perfect business sense may not meet the needs of the lady who says, "I'm not leaving my grandbabies."

Then there was a major push by overseas firms. I think I got 153 proposals from groups in India, all anxious to do the TPA work much cheaper. It absolutely bombed -- I don't think anyone showed interest. The reason was because on the TPA side, they like to keep things close at hand and because of the need for compliance, it doesn't take long for something to fall through the cracks. On things like stop loss, for example, there's so much now that is built into the system and so many other parties you have to keep happy. I have watched the overseas medical providers. They bend over backwards to try to accommodate the wants and wishes of patients and their vacations. And their facilities are top notch -- you're not going to some jungle hut. I think that they have certainly done their share. Some have also made the outreach to designate facilities in the U.S. for follow-up care. So I think that the effort has been done above and beyond the call of duty. But is that enough to get you away from your grandbabies? Also, I think employers are a little shy to promote anything that's out of the norm. It goes back to the early PPOs. I know that when they first came out, the lawyers were going nuts. They were saying, "NO, NO, NO! Don't do that! People will sue for millions of dollars and claim they wouldn't have gone to that quack if you didn't make them." As a result, the employers tended to be sensitive.

I think one of the things that is interesting is that employers -- from those covering 100 lives to those with 3,000 or 4,000 employees -- may not know everyone's name, but they do know their space or have seen them in the parking lot. There is a sense of paternalism, in a nice sense, and we have often found that employers will say, "WOW! That's great. It would save me money, but I'm not sure if my employees are ready for it."

It's like Health Savings Accounts (HSA). Employers think they are great and would love to have it for themselves. But they are not sure if their employees are ready for it or that they have the money-management skills to handle an HSA. There is a sense of protectiveness on the part of employer, and a lot of psychology on the end of the consumer that needs to be overcome.

MTT: Do you think that with health care reform and the economic pressures on employers that they may be changing their tune a little bit with regards to medical travel?
FH: I think that this is a lob in the air. There's nothing jumping out telling me that it's going to change on the medical travel issue. The key thing is going to be the impact of reform on compromising access to care and the restricted availability of doctors and providers of medical services. I think that's going to be the driver. It's going to be something like: "I have friends in Canada. He was injured this winter and his wife finally got an appointment for an MRI in JULY!!"

What I think is going to happen with employers is this: There's going to be less of an issue over cost and micro managing the coverage. I don't mean to downplay the issue of cost. But it's comparable to losing the use of an important piece of machinery and needing to get it back online as soon as possible. So if it means getting an injured or sick worker on a plane to Singapore — and getting the surgery done in a week vs. waiting a long time to have it done — I think that this rapid access to care could change things. I think that could to be the new dynamic.

MTT: With physician shortages looming, which destinations outside the U.S. are most likely to succeed?
FH: I think in terms of psychological advantages. The shortest airplane flight and the best perception of cleanliness are primary. Right now with all the issues in Thailand -- and I don't make any pretenses of really understanding the politics, if somebody said, "I can give you a great deal in Thailand," I would be hesitant.

In speaking to people about medical travel, I've learned that some of the most sophisticated medical facilities are in places that the average American thinks are dirty, dusty scenes. Clearly, marketing needs to be done with respect to those places where there are issues. I don't know the exact focus of the message, but those who are in the business should understand the problems and address potential concerns.

MTT: Do you think people will go to places like South Korea or Brazil?
FH: I don't know. I mean I think once something catches on; people will go no matter what. For instance, there are a couple of great restaurants in a part of town where you wouldn't normally go. You hear you MUST go, and all of a sudden it's got standing room only. You know its funny because I'm old enough to remember that if you had asked the average American housewife in the 1950s, 1960's, or 1970s, "Do you want to drive an SUV?" -- the answer would be NO! They would say, "You're crazy." The point is that perceptions can be changed.

MTT: What about those who don't have insurance?
FH: If they are savvy -- then yes. One of the things that I discovered — and it's sad —is that most people who don't have coverage shift their attention to getting the job for free. For whatever reason, they feel that someone should take care of them and say, "You mean I have to pay for it?" One of the things is that the younger population will get on a plane and go anywhere anytime to take advantage of a less expensive option. They are more attuned to this, I think.

MTT: Would people who are sick and need care be willing to wait?
FH: What I think is that if I am in one of the exchanges, I don't want to wait and I am willing to leave the country for care. I'd also want to know if the exchange would pay for it? I'm willing to go to Brazil or somewhere else, and I think the government will go for it — for whatever reasons.

MTT: If you had to give any advice to your constituents and TPAs, what would you tell them about medical travel?
FH: I would say to do the educated thing: Preempt the human psychology part because that's the biggest issue. That would be the same advice to the centers of excellence and all the other programs; you have to make it so it's not punitive – medical travel is a good thing.

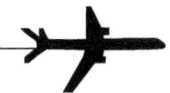

Todd E. Archer
President
Mutual Assurance Administrators, Inc.

October 2010

Nationwide, HCAA members include third party administrators (TPAs), insurance carriers, managing general underwriters, audit firms, physician hospital organizations, broker/agents, human resource managers, and health care consultants. HCAA was formed in 1980 as the Independent Administrators Association, a California-based not-for-profit that acted as a legislative and regulatory advisory group for TPAs and related service providers. Following the passage of ERISA and similar laws, third party administrators needed a voice in Washington as well as educational opportunities with leading experts in the industry. For over 30 years, the Health Care Administrators Association (HCAA) has supported third party administrators through educational opportunities from leading industry experts. With the 2010 passing of health care reform legislation, HCAA has also committed to take a leading role in legislative advocacy, working to increase its influence with policymakers and the media in order to transform the TPA industry and its role in health care.

Medical Travel Today (MTT): Please describe your organization and its market growth.
Todd Archer (TA): HCAA identified a special need in the marketplace: to provide an educational forum for the third party administration business – a place to help TPA's optimize their business activities. There are no books or manuals on this subject. HCAA helps to promote collaborative discussions for best practices, not only amongst ourselves but also with various business partners that participate in getting the job done. I think the organization has done a tremendous job of facilitating that educational process, and I think that is what is driving our continued growth and success. We continue to help TPAs identify ways to improve the job that we do for our clients.

MTT: The TPA sector has been undergoing some changes and now they are playing an important role in the development of the medical travel market. How do you see this unfolding?
TA: The term that I've used is medical tourism, the concept of traveling predominantly overseas for medical services at a much lesser cost than what you can access domestically. I also know there are one or two companies that have pursued a domestic medical tourism model, predominantly to help combat a preconception in the employer community that somehow the care that is being delivered overseas is not of the same caliber – or perhaps represents some liability issues that they are not comfortable taking as it relates to care that's received inside their employer-sponsored medical plans.

I'm familiar with the concept, but I think the adoption has not been nearly at the level that the medical tourism industry would like to see. Part of that challenge is a need for additional education as to the liability issues. I think a lot of employers get hung-up on these.

Employers also have to deal with the logistical issues. When someone is thinking about traveling to access care for a particular procedure or surgery, there are obviously other considerations that come into play. The normal logistics for travel become even more critical—having a boarding pass, hotel confirmation, transportation, and all the normal stuff we do when we travel. You have to make sure that every detail has been addressed.

I think there's also an overall sense that this may be more complicated or that there may be quality issues associated with the care overseas. Employers are concerned about how that might affect an individual on a very personal basis. They still wonder if they may be held liable if there is a bad outcome as a result of sending this member to another country (i.e., Taiwan) for this medical care. I think that more than anything this is what has slowed down the adoption rate in the employer market place.

MTT: Do you think that your organization would want to take a bigger role in that education, and is there a way to do that?
TA: Certainly. Obviously, the way the system is set up right now, most TPA's — the vast majority -- work through the brokerage market and independent insurance brokers and consultants. That is basically the distribution channel, so it's really a multi-level education process that starts with the TPA.

TPAs tend to be the quarterbacks of these plans, and everything more or less revolves around them. I think it starts with the TPAs, and the next level would probably be with the broker, which is typically the next layer that most often times sits between the TPA and the client.

Even if the TPA is a believer, the broker still needs to be educated in order to become a believer and understand how this innovative approach would benefit his or her client. Then you have to educate the client on how it would benefit them; and then you have to educate the others such as the stop-loss carriers.

Each stakeholder has to be convinced that there are sufficient savings to generate some discounts that might go toward helping fund that cost containment initiative with the client. They often say, "Am I getting any discount off the specific coverage as a result of putting this in? Is there a tangible benefit or indication that there is value to the product?" There needs to be multi-level education in order to drive the adoption rate of the concept.

MTT: Are there any particular medical tourism companies that you think are standouts as far as working with TPAs?
TA: You know, I am not that familiar with the players. I'll be honest, being located in the middle of the Midwest, and particularly in Oklahoma, we typically are not innovators. Usually, this type of new program is more accepted on the East and West Coasts. That's the case with medical tourism. Companies are not beating our doors down and saying that this is what the opportunity is. I have seen articles and advertisements, and I know that there is at least one industry conference. I am sure there is more than what I've observed, but I would not be able to list even the top five medical tourism companies out there. We did talk to a couple of the domestic companies a few years ago, and I think there are others in the market now.

MTT: Do you think that the domestic approach is more attractive right now?

TA: Again, my perception as someone who has been on the fringes and not intimately involved is that there are less hurdles to jump over with a domestic tourism approach as opposed to sending them overseas. I think it'll be an easier sell to the employer because it eliminates a lot of the perceived liability issues. I also think there are probably opportunities for some domestic providers to utilize excess capacity, especially when they have no other avenues to try to increase their patient load. This certainly gives them the opportunity to do that, and so I think some of your more progressive thinking providers will view this as a valuable business option.

MTT: Do you think that with health care reform and economic pressure on employers that they may be changing their tunes?
TA: What I see is that when these new models pop up, some folks push back. They just try to make sure that their plans stay in compliance with the new rules, which tends to eat up a lot of resource. However, cost pressures do soften the employer appetite for adopting this type of innovation.

Obviously the down side of health care reform is that it poses a lot of additional regulatory hurdles, the costs just keep escalating. That's what is going to drive employers – finding ways to balance their budgets.

Long term, as some of the costs associated with the reforms are being implemented -- and as those costs start hitting plans—you will probably see a higher appetite for cost management strategies such as medical tourism.

MTT: So this is going to be a cost decision rather than an access to care issue?
TA: Almost everything that relates to benefits becomes a cost benefit analysis at some level.

MTT: While we hear that sentiment, if you have to look at access issues and physician shortage, what destinations outside the U.S. are most likely to succeed?
TA: Puerto Rico, for sure, since many consider it to be a domestic destination. A lot of it depends upon the political environments in a given area and the perception of how American friendly the local population is. Some people perceive certain destinations as anti-American.

But there are many countries that have a history of welcoming Westerners and are recognized as a place where one can go and enjoy a visit. An example is Mexico. People say, "Go to Mexico. It's a lot cheaper and it's a nice place." Historically, I'd say Mexico would be a natural. But now, with a lot of the drug cartels and some of the things that are happening in the cities, many people don't really want to go to Mexico. The point I am trying to make is that the decision to travel for medical care might depend upon what is going on in the particular country at that particular time.

MTT: How do you feel about places like Costa Rica, Brazil, or the Caribbean Islands?
TA: I haven't really thought about Brazil. I am not a squeamish traveler and I don't worry about what might happen to me and that kind of thing. Brazil would not pose a problem to me.

I think the bigger point that surfaces here is that a lot of medical tourism decisions will depend upon the destination itself, and how much promotion there is, in general, by their tourism departments. Those companies and countries that are seeking medical tourists need to make an investment in advertising and marketing to people in the States. They need to drive demand for their destination vs. traveling to some other country.

MTT: Do you think the length of travel is a factor?
TA: I've been overseas a few times. But when you're looking at traveling with a medical condition, the notion of being on a plane for eight or ten hours can be a little bit of a chore -- especially when you don't feel well. To me, the ones that are easiest to get to and don't require a huge ten-hour plane ride would have a leg up.

MTT: What about the people who don't have insurance? Do you think medical travel has more appeal to that population?
TA: You know, that's actually a very good question. In those instances, I think it would be a matter of having a desire to travel. The younger crowd is also likely to have a more global view of the world and might be willing to take a trip to a particular destination.

Younger people may say to themselves: "If I have this done locally, this procedure could cost me $5,000. But if I go overseas I can get it done for about $1,200 — and take a vacation." They might be more willing to do this and it might be worthwhile to target this age category. You probably could use the social media outlets that exist today to try to drive a working knowledge of the product and the benefits. This might be a quicker avenue for uptake as opposed to the employer market that may take longer.

MTT: What about people who are sick but are covered by an employer that is working with a TPA—but there is a compressed access to care with the new reforms? Do you think people are willing to wait or are they willing to take advantage of this opportunity to get care faster?
TA: That's probably the one example that would drive adoption. Generally, employers that perceive a desire for a benefit or a gap that needs to be filled in their population will respond. The bottom line is that employers value employee satisfaction with the benefits package and most regard this as a business resource that is worth maintaining.

The point I'm trying to make is this: if employees express a desire to go overseas to get a procedure done, that would probably drive the discussion quicker than the TPA or broker approaching the employers and trying to sell them something. If the employer sees that there is a built-in demand in their employee population for this type of benefit, adoption will be a lot quicker then any of us can accomplish.

By and large, when employers perceive that employees are welcoming of a benefit they will regard it as something of real value. Obviously, most of them are going to look at their options to see if they can fill that demand and may perceive medical tourism as a way to save money. With the employer buy-in, it would be a win-win and that would be probably the quickest way to begin adoption.

MTT: If you had to give any advice to your TPAs what would you say about medical travel?
TA: As I've mentioned, there probably is a knowledge gap among TPAs regarding medical tourism. They will want to know who the leading players are and how to differentiate the good solid ones from the marginal companies. What are the things you

need to know about a company you might be considering that indicates that it's offering a good quality product versus one that might not be?

These are the kind of things a TPA will need to know. They need to ensure that the medical tourism company is familiar with a given marketplace, what are the "do's and don'ts," and what protocols are appropriate. Like everything else, you have to do your homework and then try to find a partner that can help you communicate a value proposition to your employer group and how it can benefit them.

MTT: Do you think your association would be open to doing something like that?
TA: Yes. We do a few conferences annually and maybe it's something we can look at; perhaps, we could run a track on medical tourism and how it benefits TPAs. This could be one of the topics at our bi-annual conference. That would be something that we can look at. What we do is set up a committee for each of the events and they go through the topics they want to present.

MTT: One final question: would you ever consider going outside the U.S. for medical care yourself?
TA: In all honesty, I don't require a lot of medical care. But at this point, it would be on my mind and I don't know that I would be necessarily opposed to medical travel. Travel doesn't really bother me -- I do a lot of it personally and professionally. My biggest concern is understanding and knowing the quality that I would get if I went overseas and what the cost differences are.

As I mentioned earlier, some of the comments were a little personalized. I would need to know that quality issues have been addressed. Sometimes it's difficult to know about domestic providers much less international medical providers!

There's got to be an education process in place. People need to be comfortable that when they travel to a given destination they are going to get at least as good a level of care as what they can get if they stayed home. Part of it is that they don't really have any qualitative measures to know comparatively the level of care they are currently getting versus what it can be.

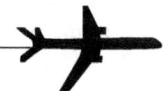

Jon Linkous
Chief Executive Officer
American Telemedicine Association

November 2010

Medical Travel Today (MTT): **Please describe the role of telemedicine and its growing importance in the medical travel space.**
Jon Linkous (JL): As you know, the medical travel industry is expanding in many areas. Since it relies upon long distance travel, there is a significant need to reach back to the patient (consumer) from the initial point of departure, both while he or she is preparing for surgery and to help arrange follow-up care. At either end of the medical travel continuum, telemedicine plays an important role for patients, physicians, and all those involved in the spectrum of care.

Telemedicine is also a way for hospitals – wherever they are located -- to expand their referral base. Hospitals use telemedicine to go into neighboring communities, rural or suburban, and establish a presence in physician offices or clinics. These initiatives generate an increased number of referrals to the hospital, a fact that is documented and is the reason why CEO's are willing to invest in telemedicine programs even if they are not reimbursed.

The same goes for the medical tourism industry. Telemedicine offers a presence in target market areas, allowing patients to link-up with specialists, such as a cardiologist or hospital specializing in open-heart surgery. This connectivity provides important information and familiarizes the individual with the location and actual travel destination. It is an efficient conduit as well as a good partnering effort.

MTT: Tell me a little bit of how you see telemedicine aiding in the construction or development of the electronic health record.
JL: I think they are independent activities, separate but related. Certainly, the more we have electronic medical records (EMRs), the easier it is going to be for telemedicine to occur.

The interesting thing is that telemedicine has grown despite the lack of quality electronic medical records anywhere in the world. What often happens is that either the vendor companies or the providers have to create their own version of an EMR because you need that record when dealing long distance with a patient or a consumer. You need to have some medium for information exchange.

If we get to the point where we have unified EMRs, it will make the process much easier because you'll be able to export information no matter where you want that information to go. If you are at a certain clinic and you want to have a procedure done in a different location (using medical tourism), you'd be able to export all of that information to the new point of care. This will save a huge amount of time and money and improve the accuracy of all patient information.

But EMRs unto themselves are not enough. They have to be exportable. A lot of hospitals have electronic records but you can't access them because they are proprietary systems and not compatible with other platforms. The whole issue with electronic records is sharing the information -- which is a political, business, or marketing issue, not a technical one. Hospitals should be willing to open up their information and allow a patient to leave one facility and go to another facility of their choice.

MTT: Describe for me a little bit about the role of telemedicine in the follow-up care.
JL: A very important issue in the U.S. is hospital re-entry. Patients, particularly those with chronic conditions, should be monitored on an ongoing basis after being discharged from a primary care facility. This is extremely important and has very specific and measureable impact on the chances of the individual being re-admitted to the hospital. In the push to reduce re-admittance rates, hospitals around the country are looking at telemonitoring for their patients as part of the discharge process.

MTT: So the role of telemedicine could be applied not only internationally but also domestically?
JL: Absolutely. The distance does not matter when it comes to telemedicine. It could be 20 miles or 2,000 miles -- the issues and benefits are the same.

Look back to the development of the electronic stethoscope. The first stethoscope was rejected because it kept you a foot away from the patient, but now we are talking about electronic stethoscopes that are thousands of miles away from the patient. The fact is that the information is actually better and can be used just as well in terms of diagnoses and monitoring the patient. It's the same situation with monitoring domestic or international medical travelers.

MTT: Talk a little about the technology challenges that telemedicine is facing in terms of connectivity – i.e., limited or no cell service from certain areas.
JL: Cell phone coverage in some countries such as Korea or Japan is actually a lot better than in the U.S. In developing nations, specifically the Caribbean Islands, they have developed a wireless network that is incredibly fast.

In terms of communications systems, certain problems have been resolved. Many developing nations have actually leapfrogged over the developed world, which is burdened with wire line infrastructure and the need to retrofit their capabilities.

Many of the major destinations for medical tourism have good broadband capabilities – countries such as Panama, Malaysia, India, or South Korea have the capability of providing very fast broadband communications and two-way broadband communications. Telecommunications should not be an issue, but it may take some investment for the health care facilities in these locales to get access to the trunk lines.

MTT: Tell me what you are hearing about the role of telemedicine in addressing health risks associated with long distance medical travel – such as the danger of deep vein thrombosis.
JL: The most important thing is to give patients information about the risks and preventative measures.

Whenever you are dealing with complicated medical issues around patient transportation, you may be getting into some interesting areas where monitoring is required. A number of companies are providing on-board telemedicine services that are available for commercial airlines.

MTT: Do you foresee the medical travel industry growing or stagnating? Is it at maturity?

JL: It's hard to prognosticate the future. I've been in telemedicine for 20 years and still have a hard time envisioning where we will be even three years from now.

We are seeing telemedicine develop throughout the world. I just came back from Iran where I spent a few days, and they are using telemedicine with the intent to provide services throughout the country. It is just an example of the capabilities that are being developed.

We are now establishing relationships that have the potential of evolving into global medical services. If someone located in Bali needs access to a specialized pediatric cardiologist in Charlottesville, Virginia -- or, vice versa -- our mission is to ensure that telemedicine makes it possible. The goal is to improve health care access worldwide. Ultimately, we are looking to have a true international health care delivery system so that wherever you are in the world you can have access to any health care professional.

There are some technical hurdles, but increasingly, these challenges are disappearing. The problems overwhelmingly involve legal and ethical issues, and, frankly, the competitive issues that we need to deal with are still apparent. That's the area that will take the most work.

At this point, medical tourism is a novel and interesting activity that is certainly growing, and has gained market size. The reality is that it isn't yet impacting U.S. industries to any great extent. But at some point, the international competitiveness angle will come into play. One of the things that we've looked into over the last few years is the idea of an international treaty that may be required as we move forward with this area.

MTT: You mentioned legal issues. Are you referring to the area of malpractice litigation? Would a telemedicine record substantiate communications between a provider and a patient?

JL: Assuming that accurate records are maintained, you certainly will have the evidence in-house that you wouldn't have otherwise with a face-to-face consultation.

The area I'm more interested in, particularly domestically, is the point where telemedicine becomes a standard of care. We are reaching the point in radiology where any hospital that does not offer teleradiology services is going to be liable: if they cannot provide 24/7 radiology services for their patients, someone may be harmed by that deficit, and they will say that the hospital violated the standards of care for the industry.

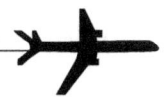

Jonathan M. Ansell
President & Chief Executive Officer
Mondial Assistance USA

January 2011

Editor's Note: *Mondial Assistance is one of the most trusted healthcare brands world-wide and has earned the confidence of business and leisure travelers seeking reliable, quality healthcare services when they are out of the country. It is also a valued resource for ex-pats living outside the US and who need to access medical care. Mondial CEO says his company is ready to serve medical travelers but questions the veracity of data regarding the size of the market. In his experience, the much-publicized volume simply doesn't exist.*

Medical Travel Today **(MTT): Tell us in your own words about Mondial.**
Jonathan Ansell (JA): For 50 years, Mondial has been helping people who travel and find that they require healthcare services to access the care they need. In 2009, Mondial Assistance USA managed 150,000 cases.

I view medical travel as a distinctly different area: it is about serving people who are willing to travel to access healthcare as opposed to those who live in a particular country or have already traveled to a location and need to access care at a local facility or an emergency room. I've seen some studies about the numbers of people that are actually medical travelers seeking care, but the exact dimensions or an accurate size of the medical travel market is unclear to me.

When you dig into the Deloitte report, which is considered the Holy Grail of medical travel, look at the source of the 750,000 base year number of travelers from which all of their projections is based. This is a key piece of information and is footnoted that the base number of 750,000 came from an Indian newspaper. The assumption is that every year thereafter, the Deloitte analysts add 20-30 percent to get to a higher number.

MTT: India is still a very popular destination for medical travel, even with the problems in Mumbai, and the cost of care in India is dramatically lower than anywhere else in the world. How do you judge quality in India or anywhere for that matter?
JA: Judging quality and then somehow guaranteeing it are the issues. If Americans want to pick up and get a hip replacement at an Apollo Hospital or a Thailand Hospital, one of the recurring questions — and one we hear most often in this business is, "What happens when there are complications or there is liability?"

Even if the patient is enticed for some reason, such as through the low cost of care, our experience is that we just don't see a lot of this traffic that everyone's talking about. We see it for emergencies and, of course, for ex-pats who are based in Thailand and Asia and want to go to a world-class facility — and there are many, such as Apollo and others.

But at the end of the day, for people to voluntarily get procedures done in these destinations because they want to save money — even if they can get over the liability issue — we just don't see a lot of activity.

MTT: It has become obvious to the marketplace that Mondial is a big player with the Blue Cross medical travel programs. Do you expect to see a significant increase in your business?

JA: Let me give you a little bit of a background. We are an international company with operations in 30 different countries. We are part of Allianz, which is the world's largest property and casualty insurance group. We provide travel and medical assistance and what we call concierge services. A significant part of what we do is to help travelers when they have a medical problem.

Typically, they fall into two categories: One is when people are on leisure travel or casual business travel and they need medical help. We have doctors, nurses and relationships with providers as well as contractual relationships with vetted providers all over the world. When these people need help, primarily for emergencies, we can meet their needs. We offer a managed care product, take risk like an insurance company, and make certain that the provider receives payment.

We organize transport to the nearest appropriate medical facility, get the patient back home and make sure to coordinate all plans with the patient's personal physician. We perform more of this type of service than anyone else in the world, particularly for leisure travelers. The second part of what we do is geared to offering these services through a number of products or client relationships that we have in place. We have our own travel insurance products here in the US as well as our other 30 businesses around the world.

As you may know, US health insurance is portable. While Americans may have higher deductibles, the vast majority of people have some sort of coverage subject to deductibles. In many other countries, there is some sort of a national health care system in place, including Canada, all of Europe and many other parts of the world. When these people are traveling out of the country, they do need to purchase some kind of policy that provides them financial protection and, hopefully, healthcare services — especially for emergencies.

We cover literally tens of millions of people around the world with products that deliver these services. These programs are pretty heavily utilized, because you've all heard stories about people who have gone on trips and had accidents or emergencies – most recently, these emergencies have occurred on a cruise ship or something of that nature.

MTT: We call them the 'Accidental Medical Travelers.'

JA: Right. This second category is where we work with insurance companies and serve their customers, subscribers, and members worldwide when they are traveling outside the country. We serve a large number of Canadians and a number of individuals covered by large US health insurers. We provide services through some of our clients that cover more than 100 million Americans. A portion of these services is designed for emergencies, but they work in non-emergency situations as well.

The vast majority of services for Americans involve non-emergent care for ex-pats who are moving overseas and need to access local medical care. We also provide a network of facilities that is available to health insurers that are performing medical travel facilitation as part of their service portfolio. As a result, there has been a lot of talk recently about medical travel, and it is a natural extension of what we do.

Today, we are able to offer people this type of service because it's very similar to what we do for those who need emergency care. We perform this service for a number of large health insurers, but again, I can tell you we see virtually no activity.

The activity we do see falls into in two categories: One is for elective, non-covered procedures like cosmetic surgery, so we have a program with a facility in Brazil where we work with the providers. The second is for dental care that people access going across border. We just don't see a lot of anything else.

MTT: Your relationships are on the business side, including third party administrators?
JA: We are effectively a third party administrator. Our activities are primarily with insurers.

MTT: Do you see more business emanating from the employer community?
JA: I think it's a very big leap of faith to ask an American, or anyone for that matter, who has access to the world's best healthcare facilities to travel to a foreign country to get a procedure that is available closer to home -- and recuperate nearer to home. Unless, of course, it's something that is not covered such as cosmetic surgery.

The current talk about why do medical travel at all is because of the cost factor. I don't see that happening unless it's for the non-covered services. To save x-thousands of dollars to get a hip replacement done in Mumbai vs. NYC is a hard sell for most people.

I recently met with a company that is representing a hospital association in Japan, and they are looking for inbound traffic to Japan. But they are not finding customers, unless the patients are ethnic Japanese who would like to get coverage there or they have family in Japan. From our advantage point, we are not seeing the demand from a cost perspective.

The second reason may be the tipping point: access to care. It may get to a point where people can't get good access to care, and that could create a different story. In Canada, they have essentially limited the healthcare infrastructure so that it covers a very high percentage of procedures that are done -- but it can't handle everything and there is a spillover. Yes, there is demand for care that isn't being filled and some individuals are trying to come over the border to get MRI's and procedures like that. There may be some demand, but I don't think it's going to be huge.

MTT: What about the patients who are looking at big out of pocket expenses, or may not have adequate insurance or no insurance at all?
JA: When you talk about the future, if the ObamaCare survives, everyone will have coverage to a certain extent.

MTT: To a degree. Think of the person who has limited financial resources: if that person needed a complete hip replacement, didn't have to pay any out of pocket expenses and could travel to a place where they've never been and be assured of the quality, wouldn't that be very intoxicating?
JA: At this point, I am telling you the truth. From our side, we're not seeing it. I know there's a lot of hype and talk about it, but we just are not seeing it. That's why we're so curious about the Deloitte study. We should be seeing at least a third of that traffic and we are not.

MTT: There are hospitals, providers and clinics that are not JCI accredited and patients are accessing care at these sites. Do you think that could account for the numbers?

JA: That's true. But from where we are seeing the global volume, it is for dental care in Mexico and cosmetic surgery in a lot of places. Both are largely non-covered procedures. I think if you look at Bumrungrad Hospital, which we know well, most of their medical travel business is coming from Indonesia, and there are also ex-pat Americans.

MTT: Do you think that travel distance is a major deterrent?

JA: Of course it is. And it's a very long trip to India and a lot of places. That's my point. They are trying to get patients from all over the world and these world-class hospitals are successful to a large degree. I'm not saying that Americans from San Francisco wouldn't get on a plane and go to Thailand or New Zealand, but the distance is always a factor.

MTT: If the insurers decide that medical travel is something they want to pursue, do you foresee that will drive the industry?

JA: It may. I suppose if the incentives were correct, it may happen. But I do still see a potential human resistance to traveling if people don't have to.

MTT: What about destinations that are closer to home, such as the Caribbean?

JA: We really haven't seen it yet. If anything, I would see the trend going the other way. I think if we have more people covered with more comprehensive healthcare benefits -- and if the affordable healthcare act goes through -- the minimum medical loss ratio requirement is going to mandate coverage. You are also going to see more people with preventive coverage. If access to care becomes an issue, then things might change.

MTT: What if there's a procedure you can't get in the United States?

JA: Then I think people would travel. If people have the resources and the urgency to get something treated that they can't get done in the US, they would travel – like alternative treatments for cancer. Look at what people are paying for things like acupuncture and reflexology; they are spending billions of dollars a year for alternative healthcare treatments that are not covered by insurance.

MTT: What are the Mondial quality standards for belonging to the network?

JA: We have a team of doctors and nurses that personally visit every provider that we work with and credential each of them. Most of the hospitals, certainly the tertiary hospitals, are JCI accredited. We have about 10,000 providers from about 1200 hospitals; and 7000 physicians and other professionals that we've credentialed and with whom we have a working relationship. We use JCI hospitals, but, we have to use others because JCI is not everywhere in the world. There are hospitals that we go out to and credential on our own.

We have another tool that is called Marco Polo. Keep in mind that we see a lot of activity in major cities around the world where people travel. Some of these cities just do not have good healthcare, so we want to get a sense of the quality of a particular hospital or clinic. That's where we'll send our medical team to do an assessment. We call this Marco Polo.

Our assessment team goes into a facility and spends time reviewing its capabilities, taking photographs, reviewing their records and, essentially ranking them on a basis of one to five. The idea behind this is if we find there's a patient that has arrived at this facility because they are in a particular location – such as Bali -- do we trust that this doctor or facility can handle this patient? It's either yes or no. If not, we need to move the patient.

We recognize that there are second or third tier hospitals around the world in countries where we have travelers. We have to understand what level of care is available -- what's good, what's not good. We need to know what the action plan needs to be if somebody has a problem.

MTT: When hospitals want to belong to the Mondial network, what do they do?

JA: We choose them. If they request to be part of the network, we put them on a list for an assessment. But we basically end up choosing them.

They can apply and then we'll send our team there to assess. Our major focus is this: can this facility treat this kind of problem? It may be a simple broken leg vs. an MI or something like that. We need to understand the capability of the facility and whether we trust them to take care of our patient.

People wind up in places like the Caribbean where the care may not be uniformly good. In those instances, we may want to get them to Miami or somewhere else.

MTT: One final question, how would you characterize your relationship with BlueCross BlueShield?

JA: We don't like to comment on relationships with our clients. What I would say is that hopefully your readers can understand the kind of capabilities we can bring to the table. So our clients hire us to help them accomplish these goals.

In the end, they hire us to take whatever coverage they are providing and make it seamlessly global. With all of the complexities of international healthcare, it's not simply the healthcare itself or paying the bill. It's making sure it's the right facility, the right doctor, and that they're connected to the local doctor back home.

Typically, there's family involved -- so it's keeping the communication lines open and making sure the payment is done. Sometimes, the patient needs to be moved, so we do a lot of medical evacuations and utilize our ambulance services to get patients to the right place.

In some cases, we've even handled terrorist bombings, or addressed the needs of patients caught in a tsunami. We sent 26 doctors to Thailand when that tsunami occurred in order to find our customers and bring them back home. We even conducted evacuations from Iraq to France. So we are virtually involved in any major sort of event or catastrophe – including the Chilean earthquake and disasters in Haiti.

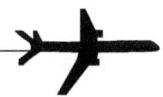

Leah Binder
Chief Executive Officer
The Leapfrog Group

January 2011

***Medical Travel Today* (MTT): Please tell our readers what your mission is with respect to helping employers and others in the payer community.**
Leah Binder (LB): Our mission is to improve the quality and safety of hospital care in the U.S. using the leverage of large employer purchasers of healthcare. The Leapfrog Group was founded 10 years ago in 2000, and we just had our 10th anniversary gala two weeks ago. It was really successful -- so we're on to our next decade.

MTT: Please share your perspectives on the medical travel industry and its prospects for the future.
LB: I think it's still in its infancy, but I think it's going to grow in the coming years. I think Americans have had it with restrictive choices among their healthcare services. They are prepared for improvements, and there is such variability in the cost effectiveness among different providers that eventually Americans will figure out that they can get far better care at a far better price if they are willing to travel a little bit.

We haven't hit it yet, but we're going to hit a tipping point and people are going to realize that there is an enormous advantage. Healthcare is so important, and it is something anybody would be willing to travel for. If you knew your child had a 40 percent likelihood of surviving a procedure at one hospital and 10 percent at another hospital, you would travel. People haven't figured it out yet. The public hasn't realized it because they don't have the information. I think as we see more transparency in healthcare reform, if it's implemented -- and Leapfrog has more measures to report – we'll have more transparency and people will begin to understand that there are some very significant choices out there to make. That's when we will see more travel.

MTT: When you say travel, do you differentiate between international and domestic?
LB: No, I don't. I think that the international travel will probably take a longer time for Americans because it is a more significant step to go out of the country. I also think there's even less information about quality of care outside of the U.S. Once there is good information, I think people will travel.

The other major trend that will impact this industry is that employers are beginning to pass more of the out-of-pocket costs on to their employees. It is rare now for health insurance to cover 100 per cent of your costs.

Nowadays, there are a lot of employers who are looking at consumer-driven health plans where they pay for a health savings account (HSA) for the employee, and then only cover really catastrophic costs. That will force consumers to shop. If you look at General Electric (GE), for example, I believe they have invested significantly in consumer-driven healthcare for their employees, so that has had a significant impact on the way employees of GE think about where they seek healthcare. They are not simply going to say okay to whatever their doctor says — they will want to know more.

As people begin to recognize that they are not simply patients but consumers, I think that the whole dynamic will change. So, again, I think that's where we are going to see more of an interest in travel.

MTT: I'd like focus on the players that you think are most well positioned to handle this influx of patients. Are there centers of excellence that you would point to or do you want to talk a little bit about centers of excellence?
LB: From the Leapfrog perspective, I would point to top quality hospitals.

We actually have a top hospitals designation, so it's formal and it's hospitals that demonstrate the highest levels of safety, adherence to safe practices, avoidance of hospital-acquired conditions and other measures on the Leapfrog survey. They need to show the highest levels of safety and demonstrate that they have the highest quality outcomes for the procedures that they perform.

Take a look at this site: http://www.leapfroggroup.org/news. Readers can review our news releases about the top hospitals of the year and the top hospitals of the decade. Since we just celebrated our 10th anniversary, we designated two hospitals as the top hospitals of the decade because they had certainly made our top hospitals list every year. We don't say we're going to designate 50 top hospitals and then go back and look at what that means. We do say, "Here's the criteria," and they have to meet these standards. Every year we raise the bar. We want the healthcare industry to improve, so we will 'up' the standards annually. When we looked at the top hospitals of the decade, the two that are cited had not simply met our standards each year, but they clearly demonstrated improvement over and above what were already considered as excellent. We felt they deserved that honor -- not just for achievement but for continual improvement.

Our top hospitals meet very high standards, and 2010 was a banner year. We were pleased that 66 hospitals met our standards, and they were the toughest standard we ever outlined. They not only had to meet safety standards but they also had to show a lower readmission rate and length of stay. So, they had to be efficient and had to have a lower rate of infection. There were quite a number of high standards these hospitals had to meet, and we were pleased to see so many of them meet them. Even among the hospitals that don't achieve our top hospital designation, you see some excellence and real improvement. If nothing else, all the hospitals that report to Leapfrog are the most transparent in the country, and transparency is the first step toward improvement.

MTT: So these were just U.S. hospitals reporting to Leapfrog?
LB: Yes. Our Board has certainly considered opening Leapfrog to other countries, but it is more complicated because the survey we do is for the coding and administrative databases here in the U.S. We would have to adapt for other countries.

MTT: Do you think that is something on your radar screen?
LB: Yes, that is something we are strongly looking at and considering.

MTT: Our international audiences would be very interested in learning about this. Tell us more...
LB: That would be great. We welcome either business leaders or hospital leaders or anyone else from another country that would like to work with us to sponsor the adoption of the Leapfrog survey from other countries.

Our Board is so interested in this because a lot of purchaser employers here in this country haven't pursued international medical tourism because they think they can't get the quality. So if you had a Leapfrog survey in place, which is what a purchaser is using here in this country, they would find it very attractive for them to consider medical tourism abroad.

MTT: How would you compare a Leapfrog survey to JCI accreditation?
LB: JCI accreditors visit the hospitals on site, which is a very intensive process that is quite resource-intensive for the hospital.

In contrast, Leapfrog dedicates 40 to 80 hours of staff time for each survey. We verify via a desk review the results of the survey, make sure they make sense, and are consistent with the other data we have for a particular hospital. We do not go on site; rather, we are a dashboard as opposed to an intensive accreditation process. We are also transparent. So most of what happens in a Joint Commission accreditation is not made public. With Leapfrog, everything that comes in our survey is made public by a hospital, and that's how employers are able to use the information to form their decision-making.

MTT: Are the hospitals that make your top list all well-known brands?
LB: No. Some of them are not so well known at all, but some of them are. There's a lot of Kaiser Hospitals on the list -- which is a well-known brand. But many of our top hospitals are not the ones that get the most PR. We are seeing that on the basis of objective evidence that a hospital is excellent -- but it just may not be known for it yet. But Leapfrog will help it to get known.

MTT: Just by having that designation?
LB: Yes – since it comes just from the data, just the reality in the data. We are an unbiased rating agency. Sometimes you'll have various rating agencies that are either driven by government entities or that have a number of stakeholders involved.

For example, what happens is this: there's a website here in the U.S. called Hospital Compare, which is run by the Centers for Medicare and Medicaid Services (CMS). It is a great idea and we're supportive of having a public website for consumers to use to compare hospitals.

The problem with Hospital Compare is that because of the way it is structured, it is part of a government agency; it is structured to meet the demands of a wide variety of stakeholders and many of those stakeholders are the hospital industry itself. So, what happens is that there's some politics involved in what they decide to report on and how they decide to show variability and differences among hospitals.

The result is that if you look at an indicator on CMS, (i.e., death by pneumonia), 95 percent of hospitals are rated as average on the national average. There's another two percent above and two percent below the national average -- but basically, everybody is average and that's because of the politics public reporting.

That is not Leapfrog. We are not beholden to a variety of interest groups. We are deliberately designed as an unbiased source of information for consumers. We report the variation as we see it.

MTT: What do you think will be the tipping point for employers to begin sending patients out of the country? When will they begin to incorporate an international medical benefit into their benefit programs?

LB: Two things: If costs continue to go up and quality continues to stagnate. If healthcare costs continue to rise the way they have been and or get worse, of course businesses will be looking for very quick answers because they can't afford the kind of escalation we've seen over the past decade. One of the biggest and quickest answers for many businesses is consumer-driven healthcare, and the more we see that, the more likely we'll see medical travel inventing the client solution.

Will costs continue to rise? I think that it could go either way. We don't know how healthcare reform issues will go, but there remains an assumption that if the federal government is unable to get healthcare costs under control, employers will pick up the excess and that's the assumption that is built into our employer-driven healthcare market in the U.S.

But that assumption is a dangerous one. I do believe employers will be looking into other options and medical tourism will be very attractive.

The second thing is quality. Employers want employees to have information about quality when they make decisions about seeking care. I think one of the hesitations that employers have to encourage medical tourism is that their employees may suspect that they don't have their best interest at heart – or that they may not know enough about the quality of care that people are being exposed to. First and foremost employers want to encourage employees to use high quality providers, and if medical tourism can help facilitate that, employers will come to the table.

Right now, employers are hesitant to say go to another state or country without really feeling like they have a trusted source of information that will benefit the employee from a quality point of view.

MTT: What can the international healthcare delivery system do to prompt this adoption?
LB: They have to prove their worth. Getting back to the quality issue, they have to be able to come up with and demonstrate an unbiased point of view that they are delivering top quality care. If they can do it cost effectively, that will make all the difference, as well.

MTT: So, cost is not the only driver?
LB: No, it is not. In fact, without high quality cost is irrelevant.

MTT: Would you like these international hospitals and providers to be in touch with you?
LB: Surely. They can email me at lbinder@leapfroggroup.org.

MTT: How much does it cost to participate in Leapfrog? Is there a fee to apply?
LB: No, we don't charge hospitals to complete the survey and report the results, and we don't charge hospitals that make our list of top hospitals. This is true for the U.S. We have not adopted this for other countries so we would have to have a different business model for other countries.

MTT: Do you anticipate this will happen in 2011?
LB: We're open to the possibility. I can't say for certain and our Board would have to approve it if it is moving beyond where we've gone; but as I've said, there is a great deal of interest on our part so I suspect there would be enthusiasm about it.

MTT: In the interim, before your Board gets on, you will be accepting inquiries?

LB: Absolutely.

MTT: What about the coding and all of the questions on the survey? Would they be adapted for each country or would they be adapted for international hospitals – say Brazil vs. Turkey?

LB: I believe it would adapted for each country. That may be more or less work, so it's hard to say. If a country is using ICD10, for example, we could adapt the survey for ICD coding. For the U.S. it is ICD9, soon to be ICD10.

MTT: From your perspective, if international hospitals participate in Leapfrog, would this obviate the need for JCI accreditation? Would it be complementary and work side-by-side?

LB: I think it would be complementary because the key issue is that we're providing transparency and that is what the employers want. They need to establish credibility in order to send their employees.

To recommend that employees go across the world to the hospital that is trusted, it isn't going to be enough to say it is accredited. That's good, but it's not enough.

They need to say, "Here's the data. Here's how they did on infection, here's how they did on mortality, and here's how they did on specific things that mean something to you."

And it's not me, it's the employer that is saying so -- it's this trusted source, Leapfrog. So, I think it's the transparency that is very valuable to employees. And that is why the employers created Leapfrog. They wanted that level of transparency.

MTT: The pushback that we're hearing on JCI from a lot of international hospitals is that they simply don't have the funds to apply for that accreditation. So, this would be a first step?

LB: Right. Exactly.

MTT: And how would Leapfrog benefit? Obviously you wouldn't be getting a fee from these hospitals.

LB: There has to be some sort of funds somewhere within the country to support the adoption of the survey, but we think that that is doable.

Putting that aside, how we benefit is this: our membership are purchasers of healthcare and they want options. This is a major option and they have asked us for it. So this meets the need of our members who are purchasers of care. That's big.

The second thing is that we think it will have a greater impact on U.S. hospitals. One of the things people said when we talked about international applications is that it will get the other hospitals across the world to learn how to get as good as the U.S. hospitals. I had to look at them and say, "I think the opposite will happen."

I think they will be embarrassed when they realize that they could do a lot better. I think it will drive our own domestic performance to compete more effectively.

MTT: What about the whole American travel tolerance index, so to speak? This seems to be a big issue for Americans.

LB: Yes, we are not good travelers. I don't think Americans have a high level of tolerance right at this moment because I don't think they recognize what is at stake for them when going outside the country. I think they think they might save some money, and so for procedures in which they might save money, you do see some people who are willing to travel. So, I'm thinking plastic surgery and IVF are often out-of-pocket costs; so if they will save so much money, many will be willing to do it.

Right now, it is driven by people who are really trying to save money. But if you get the quality equation in there, and when people recognize that a family member's life might be at stake -- and that there is such a significant difference in mortality rates or infection rates at a hospital in another country -- I think all bets are off in seeing how much people are willing to travel for that.

I don't think we are there yet, but this will have a very significant impact. If people recognize that if they go to Singapore or to South America and are less likely of getting an infection…and if the people there are nice – well, this will make the difference. I think people will travel for these reasons, but right now, they don't really understand the variation in quality that could exist even within our own country, much less internationally. But I do think once they recognize that – and that could happen very soon -- then I think we're going to be looking at a different type of travel tolerance index.

MTT: Will consumers do their own investigations regarding specific surgeries or procedures?

LB: Yes, especially with the help of the Internet. For example, we measure mortality rates for a number of procedures. One of them is pancreatectomy, the surgical removal of all or part of the pancreas, which is not exactly the most common thing in the U.S.

But the variation in costs is so significant that you're crazy not to take a look at Leapfrog before you decide on which hospital to go to for this procedure -- and the death rate can be 10 times as high at some hospitals.

We require hospitals to report individual hospital results. They cannot report for an entire system and a lot of them don't like that. We had one system that had two hospitals in their system and one of the hospitals was larger. They did a ton of pancreatectomies and they were among the top hospitals in the country for their performance – earning a four-bar rating. The other hospital did fewer of them and they were killing people left and right, a much worse performance than the sister hospital in the same health system.

So, they called us up and said something was wrong with the survey because they were the same hospital system and actually had a lot of the same surgeons performing the same procedures at these two different hospitals. How can one hospital have four bars and the other have one?

We responded that they should close the poor performing hospital to pancreatectomy procedures -- stop doing them because they are not capable of doing them well and not doing enough of them. They were killing a lot of people. It actually didn't occur to them that something was wrong -- they thought it was our data. But our data is their data – they reported this to us.

How many consumers actually looked at that data before they chose among these two hospitals? Clearly some may have lost their life over this decision. I think when people recognize that there can be that level of difference between two hospitals, even two hospitals in the same health system, they will make their own choices. A lot of people don't realize that there are differences among all hospitals and they think it's kind of like McDonalds -- and that all hospitals do things mostly the same way, with only some differences here and there. Nothing could be further from the truth.

MTT: You raise a very interesting point. There are a lot of partnerships going on now internationally where high-profile institutions in the U.S. are establishing satellite hospitals in other countries. There's obviously going to be differences.

LB: Exactly – and that's a very important point. Even the same doctor performing in a different hospital can have different outcomes. Health plans tell me this all the time.

We'll have surgeons call us and complain because they'll have some kind of incentive reimbursement to practice at one particular site -- they are getting less reimbursement when they perform procedures at one hospital rather than another. They complain, "I'm the same surgeon, but my outcomes appear to be worse in one hospital than another!"

Yes, that's true. That's because there's more to quality outcomes than just what the surgeon does or just what the doctor does. A lot of what happens has to do with what occurs throughout the whole hospital works and how the nurses function. Everything has to come together to benefit the patient -- and so when it does, it's great. When it doesn't, it can be terrible.

MTT: Are you aware of the trend among U.S. doctors forming groups to take their patients out of the country for surgery?

LB: No--I am surprised but it is intriguing. Sometimes physicians are not as transparent about their own outcomes as they should be. So I'd like to know what the patients have to go on if the physician is performing so well that people are following the doctor across the world. I think that's one of the key issues in determining the quality of care.

MTT: There has been some question about pre- and post-op care. Some patients find that when they travel out of the country for surgery they can't get access to the right post-op care in the U.S. With this model, they have their own doctor treating them before, during, and after surgery.

LB: Right, that makes sense and is very interesting.

MTT: So the bottom line is assuring quality?

LB: Yes. Our membership is employers and they have told us to start looking at this international market. There is interest, but again, I think one of the key issues as I mentioned before is that employers really need to reassure their employees that they have their best interest at heart. That means quality is their number one concern.

There is a certain natural suspicion of employers who want to send their employees across the world to save a few bucks. And that's sort of ironic since employers are spending enormous amounts of resources trying to improve the quality of healthcare in this country -- but they don't have the credibility to persuade employees that's what is in their best interest.

That's why they created Leapfrog. They needed other sources of information to show employees that they're sending them to high quality providers.

MTT: What about the safety factors and any political unrest or violence?

LB: I guess that is also something to think about, especially if we're going to work in other countries. There are a lot of considerations as we move forward.

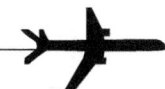

Susan Frampton
President
Planetree

February 2011

Medical Travel Today **(MTT): I suspect that some of our readers may not be familiar with Planetree (pronounced plane-tree). Can you provide us with some background on its origins and what you do?**

Susan Frampton (SF): Planetree is unique in that it was started 32 years ago by a single patient. An Argentinean woman had been in the hospital in a large academic hospital in the San Francisco area. The hospital had a great reputation and while she had a great clinical experience, she had a horrible experience on the human side of things. She felt as if she was treated like a piece of meat -- just one more item on a list of things to be checked off for the various staff that stopped in her room. There wasn't any sharing of information on what was being done or why. At the time, the traditional family visiting hours were very limited. Plus the room itself was awful -- boring white walls with absolutely nothing to look at. She came away saying, "If I got ill again I'd rather go home to Argentina where I might not have the same clinical quality but at least I'd be treated like a human being."

She decided then that it was time to change health care. In 1978 she founded Planetree with several friends and colleagues with the idea of looking at what a hospital patient experience would be like if it was designed by patients. What if they were able to make rules about how care is delivered? The mantra then and now is to make health care personal, humanizing, and demystifying for patients and families. It was really the start of the patient-centered care movement.

MTT: How does Planetree work to make that idea a reality?

SF: We work primarily with hospitals, clinics, and long-term care communities helping them to look at their practices and find strategies to make them more patient- and family-friendly. We base a lot of our recommendations on focus groups. We've literally conducted thousands of focus groups in which we ask patients 'what's your idea about the ideal patient experience?' and 'what's most important to you in the interactions you have with care providers?'

We developed a model with ten components based on the feedback we received in all those groups. These include things like access to information, compassion, patient-oriented care, and so on. One of the most interesting outcomes we're finding from using the model is that when a facility embraces the model not only do their patient satisfaction rates go up, but their clinical quality improves as well. Our model isn't just a 'nice thing to do' -- it's a solid strategy for improving care. There's a true business case for it.

MTT: Can you give us some examples of the types of improvements you've seen?

SF: Certainly. With regard to patient satisfaction, there was a study related to patient satisfaction and open chart policies. What we found was that of the over 1,000 patients who were told they could read their medical charts, nearly 90 percent were 'very satisfied' with their overall experience at the hospital compared with those who were not told. Those patients reported only a 77 percent satisfaction rate.

On the financial side, there are concrete advantages to the model. A few years ago we did a study and found that of 125 institutions using the Planetree model all reported a host of clinical and operational-level benefits stemming from patient-centered care. They cited increased patient satisfaction, increased staff and employee retention, enhanced staff recruitment, decreased length of stay, fewer medication errors, and improved liability claims experience. As we move towards a more transparent marketplace and an increase in healthcare consumerism, these are extremely important factors to consider.

MTT: What exactly is Planetree's relationship with the facilities your work with?
SF: We're a membership organization. Membership is open to any organization that's willing to commit to the mission and values of the Planetree model. There's a membership agreement they must sign. It sets expectations for the facilities and outlines our commitment to helping them implement the model. We help them develop a set of strategies to begin implementing the model.

We encourage all facilities that consider joining to visit current members and get a sense of what's involved. We also do a presentation at the most senior level to make sure they understand what they're getting into. If it's a good cultural and business fit, we move forward.

For those facilities that successfully implement the model, we provide a Planetree designation. We're hoping to make that an international accreditation standard soon.

MTT: I understand you spoke at the European Medical Travel Conference (EMTC) in Venice this year. What exactly are your international plans and interest in medical travel?
SF: We've just started to be a little more strategic in our international growth. Over the past decade we were mostly reactive in our approach. We'd get information and speaking requests and respond. Through those connections we did end up partnering in the Netherlands and Quebec to start a network of hospitals in those countries. We're now also in Japan and Brazil.

We definitely want to get our name out there as an organization that works internationally. Our appeal tends to be with higher performing facilities that are interested in patient satisfaction and customer service, which aligns quite nicely with facilities and organizations involved in medical travel. Those groups tend to have an appreciation for the values we promote. That's what brought us to the EMTC. It was a chance to tell our story and explain how we work to an interested audience.

In addition to EMTC, we've targeted a few other key conferences such as the International Society for Quality In Health Care (ISQUA) and the Institute for Healthcare Improvement (IHI). The feedback we got at EMTC was very positive so we're hopeful for those events as well.

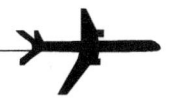

Ruth Coleman
Founder & Chief Executive Officer
Health Design Plus

February 2011

Medical Travel Today **(MTT): Tell us about your TPA business model.**
Ruth Coleman (RC): We are a fully integrated third party administrator (TPA) and have our own integrated care management company, so that is still a very important aspect of our business. I founded the company as a care management company, and we took on a claims operation when a client outsourced this function to us in 1996. And the rest is history.

We perform the full gamut — all of the claim management, reporting and analytics, care management, disease management, wellness and demand management. Additionally, we provide the other typical TPA services such as Flex and Cobra management.

MTT: Do you think the TPA industry has become a critical component of the whole health care delivery system?
RC: Yes. As a group, we tend to have a lot of flexibility, which is just one of our claims to fame. As new things emerge — as they are right now — there is a lot of opportunity.

In fact, we have so much opportunity coming our way right now that we are going to have to decide what we say no to. For every person out there, there are at least three creative ideas going on, and some of them seem to be finding us to try and do something with them. It's wonderful and all valid -- we just have to figure out what fits and what doesn't.

MTT: Where do you think medical travel fits?
RC: Let me go back and revise one thing I said. Our fully-integrated TPA clients tend to be larger than 500 employees – to around the 22,000 group size. I think some of our involvement in the travel space has to do with the fact that we tend to work with larger employers.

What we are seeing is a lot of larger employers saying that travel issues aren't that complicated anymore, and we can get our folks to the place where we believe we are going to get the best quality care at equal or better pricing. They are looking for cost controls, but they are very concerned about the quality factor. I think that quality is important to all people who look into medical travel.

The question is, "Should quality always be the lead concern?" I really only know from the larger companies that we've been dealing with that quality is certainly a primary factor. It is probably a critical factor for everybody. Nobody wants to send their employees out of the country or across the country to have a procedure done, and have them come back and say it was a nice place to visit but the quality was not acceptable.

I think of medical travel as an emerging product line, particularly domestic travel. The quality question is very important.

MTT: Maybe you can give a little more detail on domestic vs. international?
RC: I think the goals are aligned, but I do think the pricing is different. From our clients' perspectives, they are most willing to travel within the U.S. as long as they can attain a long-term financial win.

As for international medical travel, I think some of the concern is simply the distances people have to go and some of the discomfort that people were feeling about going to another country -- not knowing the language and the culture, and probably not seeing the facility and physician prior to surgery.

However, I think that with all of the fluidity in the market right now, everybody's market -- particularly the providers' market -- what we are finding is that more and more of the providers are interested in pursuing this option as a service. I'm getting calls at least once or twice a week.

MTT: When you say "providers," can you be more specific?
RC: Hospital systems, the larger ones, are reaching out. As for leaving the U.S. mainland, most people would have trouble with the travel distance and the language barrier where English is not the primary language. Traveling to a domestic hospital isn't that daunting, and we are seeing more and more interest.

MTT: Do you think domestic hospitals are responding to the competitive threats from less expensive options overseas – Asia, Caribbean Islands, Central and South America, or India?
RC: It's probably been somewhat of a wake-up call. The pricing and financial models will ultimately make medical travel viable. If employers or payers are offering a 100 percent paid benefit that includes a supporting companion that is a robust offering that is particularly appealing to somebody who has a significant financial hurdle.

What is even more interesting is that our experience is that domestic Centers are willing to look at a patient and say, "No, you don't need surgery, there's another way to treat this." That's an important part of the financial model. It's not just that I'm giving you a better discount. Preventing unnecessary surgery is a huge impact on financial outcome.

MTT: So an alternative treatment or avoiding surgery completely is being suggested?
RC: Absolutely. I think that's going to be a bigger and bigger issue because if large numbers of patients decide they are going to travel to one of the big easily recognized hospital systems -- for example Mass General, Johns Hopkins, UCLA, Mayo Clinic, etc. -- there's only so much room for discounting prices.

Part of the reason people are traveling is that when they are looking for quality they are also looking for an objective evaluation and state-of-the-art treatment.

MTT: Can you give me an example?
RC: Surely. We have had several cases where the patient was advised to undergo cardiac surgery from a home physician. We then suggested a domestic facility that would require the patient to travel. For about 10 to 15 percent of those cases, the facility has looked at the records to evaluate the patient and recommended against surgery.

In one case, an individual's physician insisted that the patient was a candidate for surgery. We requested permission to bring her in for a special evaluation to determine necessity, and the assessment showed that she was not a candidate. But somebody would have operated on her because they were thinking that she needed it. It goes without saying that unnecessary surgeries can definitely be avoided.

MTT: That's similar to a second opinion program?

RC: The intent is if the person is qualified or needs the surgery, then it would be appropriate to do so at the travel surgery center. By seeking care at another facility you are, in fact, really getting a second opinion as part of the process and accessing alternative treatment.

MTT: If you were to look more seriously at international medical travel options, which countries have the most appeal?

RC: I would say we've only really worked on the domestic side at our clients' request. I have spoken to some of the other TPAs that are doing work outside the U.S., but it's not really something we really want to get into right now.

But I think that the primary question more than anything is length of travel. When I think of someone going to Singapore for a hip or knee replacement -- which can be more than a 22-hour flight from parts of the U.S. -- the long distance travel raises concerns about issues such as blood clots. Such a long flight just increases your risk for clots, and that makes me very nervous.

And we have patients who have never been on a plane, and some who don't even have a credit card. So there are so my things to try and figure out ahead of time. Even the simplest challenge of how you're going to pay for luggage becomes a question.

MTT: How do you decide which hospitals to use? Do you have your own network of hospitals in the U.S. or do you outsource this?

RC: We do the administration for other people who are setting up the provider agreements. In the case of travel surgery, we do not set up the provider contracts ourselves.

We are seeing a combination of things. There is special direct contracting with each employer for the really big providers and employers, as well as third parties that provide the service and have set up their own networks.

MTT: How about the facilitation of the whole travel process? Do you work with any facilitators?

RC: We do this ourselves. We work with AMEX -- the travel agency folks – to set up the flights. We manage all of the rest – the stipends, the reconciliations, the tax reporting, special hotel arrangements, everything from soup to nuts.

MTT: So you're really a facilitator yourself?

RC: Yes, our nurses and specially trained customer service folks take initial calls from interested members. They ask questions since there are a few criteria that the person has to meet. This information is then passed along to one of our certified case managers who will perform additional triage.

If the person appears to be a candidate, then our staff will contact the facility and they take it from there. In the meantime, we are getting all of the forms signed and taking care of the waivers, the travel agency set-up, the stipends, and identification of hotels -- you name it!

MTT: So when the patient arrives, let's say they are flying from New York to Omaha, you would handle all of that on the ground?

RC: We have arrangements in place with the folks on the ground, including hotels, limos, and shuttles. It really depends upon the facility because what is amazing is that you'll find a lot of facilities that have thought this through and have people come in from other places to have surgery. They are more likely to have all the resources available while they are in the surgery location. We see our role as "wheels down to wheels up" to get patients to where they need to be – including coordinating care once they return home. We will coordinate care management, claims submission, disease management, and other services with their home carrier.

We are also finding that some of these folks are really difficult cases, and it's not just a question of having the surgery done well. To generate positive long-term outcomes, good disease management can be very helpful. Often, the individual's lifestyle has gotten them into some of these physical problems and surgery is not the total solution. Weight issues, diet, smoking, and other factors contribute to a chronic disease, and appropriate disease management is needed. As a result, we can get involved in providing that scope of service, although we recommend that patients stay closer to home for this to ensure better continuity.

MTT: What procedures do you find are the most sought after for travel?

RC: Heart and joint. But just today I got an email from someone seeking management for a neurologic condition. This is a first for me for this program.

I think it's really the institution and the coordination of care that matters. I've been getting my family and friends to go to these top facilities for years – and travel from wherever they are located. The medical world is really pretty small in the U.S., and so this medical travel phenomenon has been going on for a very long time in a less formal manner.

MTT: Do you think there will ever be a time where people, corporations, and employers will be looking outside the U.S.?

RC: Yes, I think they are right now. The most I hear about is India, Singapore, and more towards Asia. I think we're going to see less long-distance travel because of the airfares.

MTT: What do you hear about places like Mexico, Costa Rica, South America, Brazil, or even Panama?

RC: I haven't heard anything about those destinations, but that's probably because we're totally focused on the domestic side. I just haven't experienced it.

You know what's fairly interesting is that since we've started doing this; people call me from all over the U.S. saying they need to talk. We've been very selective in who we talk to because some of the folks we work with initially took a flyer on us managing this program. We recognize and honor their commitment to HDP.

MTT: I want our readers to understand why you think the interest level in medical travel is growing? Many are concerned that the numbers are grossly inflated and inaccurate.

RC: The question would be how much of the medical travel is truly organized vs. people just going on their own. Having a well-structured support program is a critical issue and is making it more accessible to patients.

I have actually been stunned at the interest in traveling, not just among consultants and employers. A lot of the interest is coming from medical facilities. Domestically, many healthcare systems recognize that offering travel surgery programs will make them more competitive.

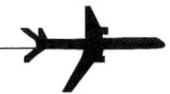

Sandra Miller
Chief Marketing Officer
Health Travel Technologies

March 2011

Editor's Note: Medical Travel Today *contacted Sandra after reading one of her postings on LinkedIn regarding recent studies on the size of the medical travel market. She noted in her post that studies which focus on numbers provided by facilitators are not seeing the whole picture of how medical travel operates today.*

Medical Travel Today (MTT): In your post you suggested that medical facilitators do not represent the whole picture of the medical travel market. Can you elaborate?
Sandra Miller (SM): Certainly. The truth of the matter is that facilitators represent very little of the actual medical travel business. In my view, they are the dinosaurs of the industry...they are not the main thrust of where medical travel comes from and they definitely don't represent where the industry is going.

In the beginning facilitators were a necessity, as nobody quite knew how to set up an international patient operations. They helped to prove the concept in some sense but as middlemen fall woefully short of what's really needed to support a true international patient program.

MTT: What does Health Travel Technologies provide that facilitators do not?
SM: We're a software and service company that serves the stakeholders. We provide them with a platform to manage all their international patient operations. We work with hospitals, hospital groups, the self-insured market, and, actually, with large facilitators.

For providers, we license our INPATRA system. Based on CRM strategies, INPATRA manages everything from lead generation, marketing and quote management to scheduling and billing. It's fully integrated and is massively scalable.

In fact, today INPATRA manages 1000 inquiries per month with no issues whatsoever, easily maintaining a first touch in ten minutes standard of re-contact. We have case specialists who work in dedicated verticals. They include doctors and RNs and specialize in cancer, organ transplant, stem cells, and so on. It's a direct-to-patient approach with end-to-end hosted business processes that serve the provider and end user, the patient, better.

On the self-insured side, right now we're working with Global Medical Conexions (GMCx) that has strong ties to helping the self-insured world make the move into global health care provisions in corporate benefits packages. Employee members will reach 500,000 worldwide.

If employers want to offer medical travel as an option to their employees, they can work with GMCx who will provide that end-to-end service to the employees choosing to exercise their medical care benefits abroad. And GMCx in turn runs its operations on our INPATRA medical travel management system, which is also accessible by the employees for health care records and communications management.

Employees lucky enough to have GMCx administering their benefits plan will find their procedures abroad are insured and backed by Lloyds of London. The warranty covers the patient's medical care in the US for one year from the time of service for any post-surgical complications that might arise.

We actually just closed the first dental traveler under this plan. An employer who just signed on with GMCx we very quickly asked for a second opinion for an employee facing an $80,000 estimate for dental work. Next week she leaves for Mexico, and her bill is far, far less than half that of the US total.

Hospital groups are another type of client we support. For example, Angeles Health International has 22 hospitals in Mexico. They've been a leader in the medical travel industry for quite a while, serving about 8000 international patients in the past couple of years, with their patient flow increasing about 30% each month.

They were finding it inefficient to try to manage – as well as pay commissions to 30 facilitators each trying to negotiate different terms and prices is just too much to handle without a CRM-based platform. They licensed our Inpatra system to bring order to the chaos and have since launched their own internally operated medical travel division.

Like many large hospitals they are simply doing away with facilitators. The lack of efficiency just doesn't make sense for them at this point – why give away so much of the revenue to facilitators? Partnering with Health Travel Technologies provides them with all the services and coordination, which is a more efficient investment than trying to develop all the necessary systems themselves.

MTT: But you also serve as a patient facilitator, correct?
SM: Yes. Our Health Travel Guides (HTG) division operates as a facilitation company and a channel for our clients and as a proof of concept for the Inpatra system that runs our sales, marketing, financial and patient case management operations. We also have Dental Travel Guides that launched in 2007 and features a large network of top dental clinics in Latin America and Asia. We handle about 1,000 inquiries a month through these different channels and that number is growing.

Let me add, too, that one of our founders, Alex Marxer, brought us the partnership of ResortCom International, where Alex was critical in the development of the CRM platform they used to manage their $400 million a year travel industry business, much of it in Mexico, helping us develop an early foothold there.

To reiterate the point that you can't always trust what you read about this industry: despite all the recent reported violence in Mexico and the whole H1N1 issue, we continue to send more and more patients there – on average more than two per day.

Now, if Mexico health care providers can grow their patient numbers amid all that upheaval plus H1N1, I think we can safely say that medical travel is probably overall is growing. Either that or the Mexican hospitals are geniuses. That could be the case, I guess.

MTT: Are you actively marketing HTG or HTT?
SM: We don't do a lot of marketing; mostly we network. Frankly, we have more potential partners than we want to deal with...we're looking to work with major hospitals that are looking to manage steady growth in international patients. Not just foreign hospitals.

We're also talking with some larger US hospitals looking into domestic medical travel options. Our system works no matter where the patient is coming from or going to. With more and more patients simply opting out of insurance and looking to negotiate directly with hospitals and providers, hospitals need a way to work with them. But hospital systems weren't built for this type of direct negotiated care, pricing or patient flow. They're built to take in walk-ins, emergencies or referrals.

With HTT, we can jigsaw in with existing systems, and make it possible for a hospital to manage its international patient systems in almost any scenario – by smart phone, PC log in or iPad app. It's an open platform that handles patient contact management, compliant electronic records upload, transfer and storage, scheduling, billing, payment, and even developing follow-up care programs.

MTT: What's your process for determining which hospitals you'll work with?
SM: We have a 9-step credentialing process for all HTG hospitals. They have to be JCI-accredited, ISO-accredited, or accredited with a similar governing body in their country or regions.

We really only work with large major hospitals that have their own standards that are higher than necessary compared to most accreditation standards. The providers we work with have relationships with the major insurers, all have sophisticated measures in place for ensure quality of care, patient satisfaction, and compliance. For the most part, they're very large institutions.

There are some small clinics in Mexico that we do work with— mostly smaller dental clinics. In those cases, the provider is already certified through an existing insurance network, for example Amexus. In addition to our own quality control measures they have to pass, these clinics are regularly vetted by TPAs representing employers, by the American Dental Association and American insurance companies.

MTT: Are you aware of other companies offering what you offer in terms of software, platform, and service?
SM: There are a few other players out there, one of which is at this moment offering itself for sale. There are some other off-the-shelf products but nothing specific to the medical travel industry like HTT. Our system is fully optimized for every aspect of medical travel – we take payment, we handle records, we coordinate schedules, transfer records, coordinate follow-up care, and so on. We manage the patient relationship from doorstep to doorstep under your brand name, delivering your brand values. We think that's a pretty big advantage.

MTT: So how does your business model allow you to realize profit?
SM: We license the technology for a nominal licensing fee that is scalable with the growth of the enterprise. Our real growth is based on patients. We take a small percentage on each patient so that we make money when hospital has patients.

It's also important to note that our case managers are salaried. They include nurses and doctors. They are not in the business of selling procedures. They're in the business of managing the relationship with the patient to ensure that all needs are met on both ends of the medical travel experience. It's an approach that ultimately serves the patient and provider better.

MTT: Where do you anticipate growth for the industry in the next 5-10 years?

SM: I think the procedures that are strong for us now—LAP band, dental, orthopedics, back surgeries, hip replacement and resurfacing, oncology, and stem cell therapies—will continue to be strong.

And treatments that aren't yet approved by the FDA in the States will surge ahead as people get more comfortable with the idea of going outside the US for care. Even once procedures get approved in the US you may find people going abroad for care simply because the doctors —say the doctors in Mexico for LAP band procedures—will have years more experience performing the procedure. So not only do you get a more experienced doctor, you save money in the process. That has appeal for many people who are paying out of pocket and facing much higher prices in the US.

But as for major drivers, we expect stem cells and cancer treatment to be at the forefront. The US follows a conventional approach to treatment; elsewhere the approach is integrative and acknowledges that removing the disease is not enough... you have to also consider the environment, nutrition, all the factors that allowed the disease to thrive in the first place. The US has been slow in recognizing functional approach to cancer and people are actively looking for alternatives. Those alternatives exist abroad.

Another growth area is the treatment of chronic disease, for example MS. The discovery of Chronic Cerebrospinal Venous Insufficiency (CCSVI) has changed the face of what we know about MS. The discovery of this syndrome was made by Dr. Paolo Zamboni of Italy. His studies revealed that MS patients seemed to have vein blockage to the brain. He tried an angioplasty balloon in the veins and had remarkable results. All those who underwent the balloon treatment (CCSVI) stopped having MS symptoms and experienced fewer attacks. We've treated hundreds of MS patients for CCSVI from all over the world and we keep getting more requests. In fact 15% of our current patients are MS patients looking for stem cell or CCSVI procedures for treatment of MS.

Although the *Annals of Neurology* published some negative findings about CCSVI—that it didn't in fact correlate to MS, and that the intervention treatment was taking advantage of patient hope —but of the patients we've worked with, everyone has had some return to function, and no one has been critical or unhappy with their decision. Obviously, more research needs to be done but sometimes patients don't — or can't, or should be ask to—wait.

Another non-FDA stem cell procedure that's gaining in popularity is being performed at Hospital Angeles Tijuana. A US company called BioHeart is using stem cells there to actually repair heart tissue damage from congestive heart failure. The Angeles center is just one of four centers of excellence they've established where people can get treatments while the FDA approval process is grinds away in the US.

Angeles is also offering stem cell therapy for the host of chronic lung conditions known as COPD for which there is no cure, but for which stem cells offer measureable regenerative effect. We think this is a very exciting growth area; stem cells are without a doubt the future of medicine.

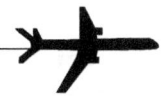

Paul Fronstin
Senior Research Associate
Employee Benefits Research Institute

March 2011

Editor's Note: *The Employee Benefits Research Institute (EBRI) is a non-profit, nonpartisan organization that studies the world of health and retirement security programs. Paul Fronstin, a senior researcher at EBRI, oversees the organization's Center for Research on Health Benefits Innovation.*

Medical Travel Today **(MTT): Tell me how your organization differs from other research groups, such as the Integrated Benefits Institute?**
Paul Fronstin (PF): We're set up like a trade association, funded mostly by membership dues. We've been around since 1978 — after ERISA legislation was passed. At the time, 13 benefit consultants, about five of whom still remain after mergers and acquisitions, got together and said they didn't' really like the way this bill was passed. They didn't know what was used to lobby for and against the bill, and they thought it was in their best interest to have an organization whose information could be trusted. Even if they didn't like what the organization had to say, at least they would be getting an honest answer.

This organization couldn't be funded solely by benefit consultants or we'd be seen as lobbying group. So, our initial funding was diversified, allowing us to retain all of the benefit consultants and welcome many large employers, unions, and trade associations. These groups represented financial service organizations that reflect the retirement side of the marketplace -- insurance companies, foundations — any type of organization interested in employee benefits related to income security issues.

We are not a lobbying group. We don't take positions on policy. We are strictly a resource for policy makers and the media for sound information, which is an increasingly challenging these days. There are different ways to influence public policy even if Congress isn't paying attention. GAO, CMS and CBO always pay attention to what we are doing, so what we do often influences what they do.

MTT: How much does it cost to belong to EBRI?
PF: To be on the board costs $28,500 annually. If you don't' want to be on the board, then you have your choice among $4,000, $7,500 and $15,000, depending upon what membership benefits you are interested in.

MTT: Are you familiar with the medical travel industry and the conflicting reports on the volume of travelers?
PF: Yes. I read the recently released report.

MTT: I was disappointed not only in the source, but also in the methodologies used. Please give our readers your perspectives and what you think is needed for more accurate research in this field.

PF: This is not an area that our members have asked us to do any work in.

MTT: Yet.
PF: Yes. Yet, we'll see if they do, but I think they'd turn more to consultants for advice because they are the ones helping them create the benefit, the plan design decisions. That's not what we really do. But, you never know.

MTT: I do think the interest level will accelerate very soon — so I would imagine that this is going to start to get on your radar screen.
PF: Yes, it may very well accelerate with us at some point. It's just not something where I can predict what will happen. But I think it's a no-brainer to explore. Employers are looking at different ways to control costs, and this is just one other tool to explore. I mean, why not? It's there.

They may have issues and concerns, and there are things they can certainly work through. It may make sense in some context, and it may not in others. Some employers are considering domestic medical travel as a first step, while others are exploring international opportunities. There's certainly no reason not to put it on the table.

MTT: What do you think would raise the employer comfort level?
PF: I think one of the biggest concerns is quality: are they truly getting the same level of quality that they would be getting in the United States for less money?

There's also the issue of follow-up care when someone returns home, either from another U.S. city or a foreign country. They can see the cost savings. It's what got their attention. But are they really getting value? That's the single issue related to this discussion.

MTT: Do you think that there's any pushback from Americans on the length of travel?
PF: Yes, to a certain degree, but I don't know what somebody's tolerance is for getting on a plane for these circumstances.

It doesn't matter where you are going, the cost of getting on the plane is the same in terms of getting to the airport and the time to security, the time to wait and the time to get a taxi, wait for your bags, etc. It doesn't matter if you go on a 30-minute flight or a 30-hour flight. All of that is fixed, and those areas seem to be the biggest sources of anxiety. There are so many choices today. I hear about options in Costa Rica and Mexico for medical care. I hear about South America and Brazil. These destinations are not that far. It's not like going to Asia.

In time, there will be more choices. How far people will travel will depend upon the choices available. If the market is there, other nearby countries will be looking to develop the infrastructure to attract people.

MTT: So which countries come to mind most readily?
PF: Costa Rica, Mexico, India, Brazil and, perhaps, Thailand.

Canada can't be ignored, either. People travel there to get prescriptions. They may not be going there to have a heart valve replaced, but people cross the border just like they do in Mexico except it's for prescriptions.

MTT: Can you weigh in on domestic medical travel vs. international travel?

PF: I believe employers have already taken that first step for domestic medical travel. If there's a center of excellence, they'll include it as part of their benefits. So whether it's sending someone to the Mayo or Cleveland Clinic, I think employers are open to it.

MTT: What do you think are the best venues for employers to present this new range of benefits to their workers?
PF: Just giving them a flyer is not going to be useful. These are people with serious conditions who are skeptical about a benefit changes. — especially if they're being sent overseas. They'll have a lot of questions and plenty of discomfort at first.

MTT: So if you were going to consult to an employer or one of your constituents about rolling out a benefit in domestic or international medical travel, what would be the steps you would take?
PF: The focus should be on the people who would be taking advantage of this. Privacy issues also have to be considered.

It's important to provide a resource, maybe even one-on-one counseling., or Even if a third party is hired to get the word out on conditions, diseases or surgical procedures, Resources must be made available to help people make decisions and take advantage of options.

MTT: What size employer groups could offer a medical travel benefit?
PF: Employers who self-insure will certainly see this as a great benefit because it affects the bottom line. There's more skepticism in the fully insured market because employers don't always realize savings in their premiums. So, it's a tougher sale; unless the insurance companies are offering incents that can be seen up front.

MTT: Do you think employers are concerned about the lack of reliable data on this industry? Would the EBRI be a resource for that kind of research?
PF: Maybe, it depends upon the scope of research. It's not something we have on our agenda, but that could change.

MTT: What would make you change?
PF: It depends on the research and funding available. There's got to be a public policy twist to interest our members; however, it might be something we think is important.

MTT: What if CMS/Medicare decided to offer an international medical travel benefit? What are your thoughts?
PF: We don't take positions on; say for example, whether Medicare should do something like that.

Should Medicare look at it? Maybe it will. And just because Medicare is looking at it, doesn't mean it is going in that direction. If Medicare doesn't look at it, it will never know what the answers are. There's never a discussion to have.

MTT: That's fair. Do you think that this is a natural fit for value-based insurance design?
PF: I do think it is a natural fit. The notion behind value-based design is to get out of the limits of a one-size-fits-all cost-sharing structure. By this, I mean where everything is covered under the deductible. The co-insurance is the same for in- or out-patient regardless of which doctor in the network is used.

There is a benefit to providing an innovative plan design to share costs and influence behavior. Certainly, if an employer wants to steer people toward a center of excellence -- that might be across the street, across state lines, across the country or across an ocean -- they can use cost sharing incentives to get attention.

MTT: If you had to give one piece of advice to this industry to help it grow, what would it be?
PF: The value proposition must be proven in terms of quality.

MTT: Is JCI Accreditation enough? What if the Leapfrog Group came up with an international survey tool? What are the quality benchmarks that employers need to hear?
PF: It's up to those organizations to develop benchmarks; for example, 30-day risk adjusted mortality rates after open-heart surgery.

Organizations must develop standards and, once they do, then employers will look at that information and determine if they are willing to send their employees to a facility in another country.

MTT: Do you think there's a need for a credible trade organization to do this?
PF: A trade organization would certainly be helpful, but I don't hear the need for one from my members.

MTT: Would the tipping point for employers be the generation of data and reporting that were coming from a reliable source?
PF: That would help. When employers share their stories, it convinces a peer to take action.

MTT: Would you ever consider going abroad for medical care?
PF: I hope I'm never in a situation to make that decision.

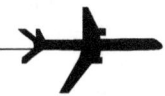

Abbie Leibowitz, M.D.
Fellow of American Academy of Pediatrics
Health Advocate, Inc.

April 2011

***Medical Travel Today* (MTT): What is your familiarity with medical travel? Do you come across it in your business activities with Health Advocate?**
Abbie Leibowitz (AL): Yes, we do. Let me take you back a bit.

I was a medical director with US Healthcare, and then the chief medical officer at Aetna U.S. Healthcare after the merger of the two companies, so I go back to the mid-'80s in this business — I'm getting old!

We've seen a modest amount of interest in medical tourism among our clients at Health Advocate — medical care delivered overseas or travel for medical services.

I remember in the late 1980s and early 1990s when, at U.S. Healthcare, we were approached by a group of physicians from Israel. They had a new procedure for knee replacement surgery. The cost for the procedure as well as a full course of rehabilitation physical therapy after the surgery – plus travel to Israel for not only the patient, but also a family member – could all be done for about half of the cost of doing it here in the United States. So the idea of traveling outside the country for medical care is certainly not a new story.

MTT: How long ago was that?
AL: Maybe 1989 or 1990. And I'm sure that was not the beginning of the story either -- it's just when I became aware of it.

Clearly, the interest in traveling overseas for medical care has been driven mostly by two factors:

One is obviously price. Services overseas are often significantly less expensive than here. The second factor is there are things done abroad that are not done here, that some people may be attracted to. These may be procedures or treatment approaches or medications that are not available or approved in the United States

So you have to look at this as either going overseas to receive care that is available here; is recognized as a good and established treatment, but is either done less expensively or better overseas; or going overseas to get care because it is not approved in the United States.

MTT: It seems like you have a thorough and long history with medical travel. How would you say it stacks up to what it is in 2011?
AL: It's certainly much better organized today. As you are well aware, it has been written about in this newsletter and elsewhere, and there are dozens of facilitating organizations working in this space. They work on a fee basis and either have connections to specific facilities and doctors overseas or just functioned as a facilitator.

The idea of going abroad for services is easier for individuals today than it was when I first got involved in managed care. Back then, you were really on your own seeking out services. If you go back to the '80s, nobody had the Internet sitting on their desk like we do today. Things have certainly changed as the ability to access these services has become much easier.

MTT: Do you see a growing interest in medical travel among consumers or employers and payers?

AL: If you judge by the great propensity of available services and the promotion of those services, you have to conclude that there's increasing consumer interest.

However, the truth is that sitting where I sit today at Health Advocate, we don't see a lot of it. We don't receive many inquiries from the 20 million people we serve.

Now, that doesn't mean people are not interested in it. Instead, it might mean they don't come to us with any great frequency. We certainly have had a couple of cases, but it's not as though people are beating down our doors to identify places abroad where they can go for infertility care or cancer treatment or a transplant.

MTT: Do you ever reach out to these people and tell them this service is available? Is your observation just anecdotal based upon their interest or inquiries?

AL: It's based upon the level of interest and number of inquiries we get, or rather don't get, from our subscribers. It is also true that we don't promote ourselves as having a lot of expertise in this space.

MTT: Would you ever?

AL: It's an interesting question. As I was preparing for this interview, we started talking about that. We have a good relationship with several organizations that work in this area, but we don't see ourselves doing it directly at this time.

If we get requests, we do have a database of facilities and physicians our subscribers have used. We can get started on the search and then call on outside resources that we can work with.

MTT: Do you foresee that there will be an opportunity in the near future to work with employers on getting them to adopt a medical travel benefit?

AL: Several years ago, there seemed to be more employer interest in this area than today.

Clearly, employers, especially large employers, who are self-insured and pay for the medical services that their employees receive, have an interest in helping their employees find less expensive care. The interest in encouraging people to get care abroad as a formal benefit seems to have waned in recent years.

There are certainly programs out there, but, today, employers seem to be focusing on other ways to reduce medical costs.

So we haven't seen very much activity in this space on the employer-side. There are still employers that offer travel benefits, but there certainly is not a groundswell of interest in this approach.

MTT: What do you think would ignite their interest?

AL: The biggest concern has always been assuring the quality of care that an individual gets, and that is not becoming much easier.

Finding American-trained physicians who are practicing abroad and who have developed programs to attract patients from the United States has become easier.

In terms of the number of patients who need medical care and leave the United States compared to the patients coming from overseas to get care here, there's a far greater influx of patients coming here for care than there are patients going abroad.

In the northern border states, there is a considerable flow of Americans going to Canada for care and there are many Canadian programs that actively promote that care is less expensive in Canada.

To a certain extent, the same applies at the southern border, where people are going to Mexico for care; although it doesn't seem to me that -- at present -- the flow into Mexico is nearly as well developed or as comfortable as it is to go into Canada to access care.

MTT: Access to care is a consideration for many people. Do you believe access would have an impact on any kind of trends in medical travel?
AL: It may, but there's plenty of good care accessible and available in the United States -- if you are willing to travel, and going to another city or state is typically a lot closer than going abroad.

MTT: You describe the domestic medical traveler.
AL: Would you say, "I can't find a physician within five miles of my home who can treat my arthritis, so I am going to go to Latvia?" I think that would be a little odd.

I don't think medical tourism is truly driven by the lack of access to services because I think anyone willing to travel overseas could certainly find a domestic provider somewhere available and able to provide that care. The other thing that shouldn't be overlooked in this discussion is that Medicare does not provide any coverage for services received outside of the United States. That cuts off a significant number of chronically ill people from this adventure of going abroad.

MTT: What about for procedures that are not available here – like stem cell or organ transplant?
AL: I would think that you could really look at the whole transplant situation, but there are some important ethical issues surrounding how organ donors are found in some countries. That's a serious concern. But transplants and the limited supply of organs in our country is one of the highest profile services for which people will travel abroad.

MTT: And cost is usually no object.
AL: To the individual, cost is often no object in these situations. But staying in the United States, using your health insurance benefits and getting a transplant here in a high quality program, is the lowest cost-option on multiple levels for the individual.

However, it is unfortunately true that many Americans die before a transplant ever becomes available. So, how do you put a price on that?

MTT: What about embryonic stem cell treatment?
AL: There is much less political overtone to some of these interventions abroad than there is in the United States. But it's my belief that the level of expert care offered in the United States can't be matched elsewhere. It doesn't mean we don't have many quality of care issues and inefficiencies in our healthcare system that can't be improved, but at the highest level of care, it's very hard to argue that the United States is not as good or better than anywhere.

However, there are definitely programs abroad that have great experience, wonderful outcomes and are doing things that cannot be done here. The challenge to the individual is to identify the level of excellence abroad -- and that's why you write a newsletter and why we started Health Advocate.

MTT: Exactly. So what would you recommend to a patient that had prostate cancer and heard about this HIFU treatment in Mexico?
AL: I would recommend they seek the level expertise appropriate to their condition in the United States, and speak specifically to that physician about all of their treatment options including those that are available outside the country.

MTT: Do you believe physicians in the United States. are giving that information to patients?
AL: Yes I do. I am sure that at the level of expertise that we help our subscribers reach, physicians are more than willing to discuss all of the various care options.

If you were to go to the top-tier academic medical centers of the country, I think you could trust the physician to give you an honest opinion about the things that could be provided outside the country that are not available here.

Typically, many of these "medical innovations" that are being practiced abroad are working their way through the approval process.

If they haven't been approved, it may be because there are concerns about the effectiveness or the safety and value of the procedure or treatment.

I think you have to be a little skeptical about care offered outside the United States I think you also have to do your research and decide whether you want to go abroad and get the opinion of the doctor who provides any one of these procedures in another country.

MTT: Can we go back to the discussion about Medicare? Do you think the U.S. government would start outsourcing healthcare to other countries – places not too far away where they are building phenomenal hospitals and delivering high-quality care?
AL: There are two answers to the question: You phrased the question to say, "Gee, why wouldn't the government do that?"

However, if you take a step back and look at the present health debate in the country relating to Medicare costs and spending, this idea is not on the agenda. So, if you ask me to predict whether or not over the next 3-4 years we would see Medicare expand to cover treatment overseas, I would doubt it very much. That's not saying whether or not it's a good idea, it's just not in the forefront of the important discussions happening today.

Medicare does have a lot of flexibility under present legislation to conduct pilot programs. Certainly, they could turn around tomorrow and say, "Let's put together a pilot and study the value of having people get care overseas." I just don't think it's on anybody's agenda right now. I think there are other priorities to address.

MTT: Do you think it's a good idea?
AL: I think it's interesting, but there are certainly challenges. I think you'd get into issues of how to credential providers and how to decide what to cover. There are a many issues around making this public policy.

MTT: Have you ever visited these hospitals outside the country?
AL: I have visited hospitals in Western Europe, England, France and Brazil.

MTT: Where did you go in Brazil?
AL: We were in Rio and it was more of a personal visit, nothing formally organized.

MTT: I think you may find it an eye-opener to visit some of these places.
AL: Well, American-style care, Western medical care is spreading to other countries. American hospitals are setting their sights on opportunities in other countries. It's very hard to get physicians to leave Boston and take up shop in the Middle East.

There is a lot of interest in spreading the flag around the globe; both the export and import of Western medicine..

MTT: Do you foresee more of these alliances and partnerships?
AL: Yes. Medicine is a big business. It's one of the best export industries that we've got in this country. We manufacture good healthcare and we export it abroad. It drives money through multiple levels into our economy.

If you're the guy walking down the street in Beijing who has cancer, you deserve the same expert level of treatment that the person walking down the street in Baltimore does.

MTT: So if you were invited to go on one of these healthcare missions, to South Korea or Brazil or one of the healthcare destinations of excellence, would you go? Would you entertain that?
AL: I'd entertain that if I thought that it would be helpful and consistent with the business that we're in at Health Advocate.

MTT: Is there anything we didn't cover about medical travel that you think we should touch upon?
AL: I know that the focus of the newsletter is medical travel, but I point out that there are many innovative programs happening here where employers are focusing on quality medical services available to their employees and facilitating the employee's transport and travel to those facilities.

Lowe's Home Centers is a Health Advocate client. They just put together a relationship with the Cleveland Clinic and we are part of facilitating its electronic second opinion service and helping employees access travel benefits.

So, there is awareness among employers that good care is valuable even though it may not be less expensive to get heart surgery, for example, done in Cleveland compared to having the procedure done in another community hospital.

But there's a focus on the quality and outcomes of the care, so Lowe's and other employers are attempting to channel cases to places that have better results.

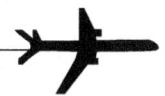

Stephen B. Bonner
President & Chief Executive Officer
Cancer Treatment Centers of America

April 2011

Editor's Note: *Readers in the United States are no doubt familiar with the Cancer Treatment Centers of America (CTCA) thanks to their successful advertising campaigns. But their reach goes well beyond the shores of the United States. In fact, in 2010, CTCA received more than 10,000 international inquiries.*

***Medical Travel Today* (MTT): Give our readers a little bit of a background about you and how you got started at CTCA.**
Steve Bonner (SB): I am the president and CEO of Cancer Treatment Centers of America and have served in this role since July 1, 1999.So, I'm coming up on 12 years. I'm a lawyer who really grew up in financial services and worked for several companies — starting businesses, introducing new lines and doing some turnarounds. Along the way, I was introduced to Richard Stephenson, the founder of CTCA, and, after two years as a CTCA Board member, I stepped into the CEO role.

I came here because I think it's a really unique offering in healthcare, and oncology in particular. When Dick created this company in 1988, he was at least a couple of decades ahead of the market in his vision, and I thought the market was moving toward the CTCA vision of patient empowerment, and a holistic and integrated style of care.

Dick Stephenson was motivated by a personal experience: His mother had cancer. Stephenson is a globalist and an international merchant banker who was able to find an array of promising therapies that could have helped his mother, but could not get the healthcare bureaucracy to try or even listen.

Sadly, his mother died and, in his opinion, hers was an unhappy and untimely death. He believed that no one's mother should be subjected to that, so he created CTCA. By the time I came, the organization was about 10-11-years-old; it had grown to a certain level, but was not growing much.

I was attracted to how unique the company was, the value I thought it offered to patients and how it might help change some of the unhappy parts of the American healthcare system. I also spoke with patients who had come to CTCA and, when I looked them in the eye and they said if it wasn't for CTCA they wouldn't be here ... I felt compelled to join them. Specifically, to offer life-saving hope and healing options to patients who say they can't find elsewhere -- and then to add more talent and technology to improve continuously.

And that's a pretty unique opportunity to have in this business.

MTT: I would say that could drive anybody to do business.
SB: We just boasted about this at our quarterly meeting with the Center for Health Transformation, the organization Newt Gingrich founded. CHT membership met at our CTCA hospital in Phoenix.

We always start important meetings with a patient of ours telling his or her story. The woman who talked to the group yesterday said before coming to CTCA she had been told she had six months to live, was undergoing horrible chemotherapy and was not effectively managed or communicated with. She came to us in January 2010, expecting to die within the next five months.

Yesterday, 14-months later, she stood up and told us she is actually cancer-free. We seek to do good business. We can create a lot of great products, jobs and economic value, but to be in the business of saving lives and now innovating healthcare is a great place to be. As you say, it could drive anybody to do business!

MTT: I would say so. Congratulations! Let's talk about the medical travel industry, how you see the industry growing and what part CTCA would play.
SB: I think we're significantly into that market today if we define medical travel as healthcare consumers who have to leave communities to find services they value.

Today, while we don't see that much international travel at CTCA, our average patient travels 514 miles one way to come to us for care.

MTT: Five-hundred-and-fourteen miles?
SB: Yes! Obviously, they are all driving by their own community oncology offerings. Many of them bypass Mayo, MD Anderson and Sloan Kettering to get to us.

Individuals stay with us for extended periods of time. In order to serve them, we don't simply offer cancer treatment facilities. We have guest quarters that we built as a part of our centers and we have relationships with local hotels and "Bed and Breakfast" places that provide access and knowledgeable support about hosting cancer patients.

We also have cars, limos, shuttles and drivers that move patients, pick them up at the airport, bring them to the hospital, take them back again and also make dining, recreation and shopping available while they are with us. So in the travel business, I know we're very active. We see quite a few patients from Alaska and Hawaii and the Caribbean islands, for example.

Internationally, we host a fair amount of information-seekers on our Web site, but we have still only seen just a trickle of patients.

MTT: Have you gone after them? Have you marketed to the international community?
SB: No, we haven't, other than on the web, of course. That is a growing interest for us, especially since we are seeing so many of them on our website.

We have just done a fresh analysis of international medical tourism. I think we've done a good job of sizing the market of both inbound and outbound patients, although the research we did reflects some wild disparity among the experts in terms of how big this market is.

MTT: Who did your research?
SB: We assembled research from DeLoitte and McKinsey, and also from the Bureau of Economic Analysis and from the Office of Economic Cooperation and Development (ECD). Just looking at the estimated annual inbound medical tourists to the United States, the research pointed to a range under 100,000-400,000 annually. The outbound ranged from almost nothing, according to McKinsey, up to almost 1.5 million, according to ECD.

MTT: There's a lot of discussion in the industry about those numbers and what is real. One of the questions is how is medical travel reported? Does CTCA record the patients coming from another state or another region of the U.S., and do you really track that number?

SB: Yes, we sure do. Part of our founder's vision for making sure we were patient-centric was to not let government bureaucracy; hospitals or doctors get in the way of innovation. That is what we're built upon — almost a pure direct to consumer model. We think of ourselves as the most active advertiser in the non-pharma sector of health-care, and certainly in the hospital sector.

As a result, if you have studied us, you'd see us behaving very much like a traditional direct marketer. We advertise, we track media and our messages and match that to our response from initial inquiry to arrival of a patient.

We obviously then track them geographically because we want to match our advertising activities to media placement to geography. We want to know what is working and what isn't.

MTT: Good for you. How many patients do you treat annually, and would you say that you're a court-of-last-resort for these patients or is it the first choice?

SB: We're hosting about 4,300 new patients each year and that's been growing about 20 percent annually for the last several years. We're probably seeing around 12,000–14,000 patients annually, which would be the new patients plus those returning. We hope we are the court-of-last-resort and that none of our patients need to seek another court of higher jurisdiction. Our average patient is diagnosed somewhere else, they're treated on average two other places and then come to us. We hope they find lots of reasons to stay in our care.

So, they are very savvy, experienced and generally unhappy with the care they've received by the time they arrive. We also tend to see later-stage and complex cancer patients largely because of the way the market works. So to stay with your analogy, in about 1/3 of our patients, we are the first court; for 2/3 we take appeals from other providers.

MTT: Can you describe the typical process a patient goes through to choose a cancer hospital?

SB: A patient begins with a terrifying cancer diagnosis from a trusted family physician, who says, "Go to Dr. Smith, she's my oncologist." The patient has a pretty strong instinct to keep these relationships intact and do what their doctor tells them.

Off they go, and they don't even think about CTCA or other alternatives, and they get treated by Dr. Smith. If treatment works, that's fine and they are all happy and they go about their lives. CTCA does not enter the picture.

Typically, it's when treatment doesn't work that they start looking around for options. I should note that even this time-honored process is changing. Today, even the first referral is considered more carefully by the patient. When they come back to their diagnosing physician for a second visit, the patient knows more about the disease than the referring physician.

Patients and their families are on the web, in their networks and they're looking, and we see them on the web site we host. There are more than 8 million unique visitors each year on our web site.

MTT: Is the web becoming even more important in this process of finding the right care?

SB: Without any doubt. The quest for information — national and international — is certainly exploding in oncology. Our data says that around 10,000 international inquirers visited our web site in 2010. We have people staffing our inbound phones 24-hours-a-day, 7-days-a-week, including oncology information specialists who can talk with patients and chat with them over the web. This allows the patient to discover information without coming here. They learn what we offer, and what it might add or not add to the care that they have received.

They then decide to come. But because of the prevailing relationship-driven, community referral-based model in healthcare, we don't usually see patients early in their disease. Generally, when care is not going well and they are losing hope, they look to the horizon for hopeful options. That's what we restore ... hope.

Often times, hope has been taken away; like the woman I mentioned in Phoenix who thought she had no alternative but to prepare to die. She was writing notes for her children to open on their birthdays, when they got their drivers' licenses and so on. She came to us and we offered legitimate and hopeful options that are working.

MTT: Do people talk to you on SKYPE on the international level?

SB: Not to my knowledge, but we do have growing video confession tools. And we are becoming more active in social networking.

MTT: When you market directly to consumers, does that encompass employers?

SB: It does. Increasingly it does.

MTT: In what way? Tell me something about your relationship with employers.

SB: We have a team whose sole responsibility is to get out and talk to employers who are looking to buy healthcare intelligently in this burgeoning environment of wellness investment. In this health transformation, we know more and more major employers are buying healthcare directly, and we are participating. We have people that are out presenting CTCA to employers, and we do have direct contracts with employers.

MTT: What we hear from the marketplace is that employers and payers are looking for quality benchmarks, and that's what may be missing from some of these international hospitals – they are not willing or able to report outcomes. Are you able to report outcomes?

SB: You're touching on one of our favorite subjects.

Patient access to comparable, reliable results is a huge deficiency in healthcare today, and that information will be a cornerstone for a high quality, a low cost healthcare system. As we move toward a more patient-empowered system, all of the sudden we will see a more disciplined healthcare market, the way it is in every other consumer-driven market. But, to get there, we've got to provide the consumer reliable, accessible, easy-to-understand information to compare among the different services that are available. We feel compelled to do this.

We have been tracking our length-of-life outcomes and publishing this data on our web site for a couple of years. We believe we were the first in oncology to do so. We also study quality-of-life, and publish that data on our web site. Finally, we study patient experience, using survey instruments that allow us to watch on a daily basis what is working and what isn't, and to be able to fix things that aren't working to perfection.

MTT: What tool do you utilize?
SB: Bain & Company developed a "Net Promoter Score technology," and it's the most rigorous measurement of patient loyalty we can find. It's an 11-box score platform. The top scores indicate that consumers feel so strongly about the experience that they want to go out and actively promote the service to others they know.

The top two boxes are promoters, the bottoms six are detractors and the others are neutrals. We run the survey, total the top two boxes and subtract the bottom six boxes. That gives us a "net promoter score." About three years ago, Bain wrote a book that said the CTCA consistently produces the highest net promoter scores of any company they have found in any industry that they have studied. And we publish that data on our web site, as well.

MTT: Are you working with other industry providers to promote this type of activity?
SB: Yes. We're putting together a coalition led by a trusted consumer research organization and supported by oncology providers like us to conduct consumer quality research.

The goal is to define what quality means to the consumer, and we envision a component on the patient, their family members and their employers to really understand how they define quality.

We're assuming that length-of life, quality of life and the patient experience are reasonable proxies for this measurement, but we're trying to move the industry to let the consumer teach us what quality means to them --and give them reliable metrics to select the best provider ... for them.

MTT: Are you familiar with the LeapFrog Group? Its CEO Leah Binder told us a few months ago that they were going to be coming out with international ratings for hospitals. How would you think you'd stack up against Albert Einstein in Brazil or Bumrungrad?
SB: We're very active participants in the LeapFrog Group. It will be interesting to see.

Leah Binder also says that they promise to come out with oncology-based measurements rather than lumping all of the hospitals together. We know Leah very well, we have great admiration for each other and we cooperate well together.

We want to help LeapFrog get there because, right now, measuring oncology quality against quality in GYN or general surgery is not very meaningful to patients, employers or insurers that are looking at us.

MTT: What about pricing? Can you compete for the medical traveler?
SB: Yes. After reliable quality information, price is the next critical piece of the equation. An empowered consumer needs pricing information, and that's virtually impossible to get. We're as weak as anyone in dealing with this issue today.

But we've taken on that challenge, and we're close to coming to market with a guaranteed array of comprehensive services and a guaranteed price for the evaluation phase of care. In the next two years, we've committed to the delivery of guaranteed prices for the treatment phase, as well.

Once the consumer has that kind of information, they can do what they do in high quality industries: shop for price and value. They can look not only nationally, but also internationally; and make a much more informed judgment about where the quality is, where the value is, and where the price/quality combinations lie. They will start to buy accordingly, like they already do under Health Savings Accounts and in self-pay segments, such as Lasik surgery.

MTT: Would you say that you provide treatment or procedures that can't be found anywhere else?
SB: I would say that we offer a combination of therapies that can't be found anywhere on the highly integrated, under-one-roof model that we offer. As you can imagine, if you're in oncology and your dominant customer has complex cancer, then you've got to have the most sophisticated traditional therapies including radiation, chemotherapy and surgery. We have that. We need to offer those traditional therapies that treat the tumors. Since the core of the problem resides in the immune system, we must support the immune system ti re-engage it to battle the cancer. But there is also the double-whammy that traditional therapies also tend to assault and further debilitate the immune system. So, we surround those traditional therapies with what we believe to be the most intense nutritional support that can exist in any cancer facility. We add to that naturopathic support, the mind body connection, spiritual support, exercise, pain management, acupuncture, massage, chiropractic, humor therapy, laughter therapy, pet therapy ... and on and on. We see architecture and environment as part of the healing process. So our centers feel and look more like hotels or spas than hospitals.

MTT: You have chiropractors?
SB: We sure do. We have full-time chiropractors on staff in our hospitals, and we have wonderful relationships with the chiropractic community that we continue to invest in. Chiropractors are a wonderful group of healers and are greatly valued by our patients, their family members and our stakeholders.

MTT: Now, I have a $64,000 dollar question for you: Are you building outside of the United States?
SB: And the $64,000 dollar answer is: not yet.

MTT: Are you partnering with anybody outside the United States?
SB: Yes. We partner with researchers and innovators in other countries, but not as robustly as we'd like.

MTT: Is that something that you would find intriguing?
SB: Yes, we absolutely would. Our founder has extensive experience offshore and is very comfortable doing business outside their. A few years ago, we looked at the healthcare city Dubai is building. We were intrigued by the possibility of being their specialty cancer provider, but decided we didn't know that market well enough and we still had a lot to do to build our footprint in the United States. So we passed. In the United States, we are now four hospitals; at the time we looked at Dubai we were three hospitals. And we just made another commitment to break ground for the fifth in Atlanta, where we expect to open next year. We're looking at other expansion opportunities in the United States. We've just done a fresh analysis on the international market, both inbound and outbound, and we're curious.

MTT: So if Dubai is not the right location, are there any other areas closer to home that would be more appealing? Everyone is talking about the Caribbean, Central America and Brazil.
SM: We've actually seen a trickle of patients from the Caribbean, but not significant. Certainly, the proximity to the United States and our familiarity with some of those islands will draw our attention.

MTT: So inbound medical travel from that region is also of interest?
SB: Yes. Basically, many patients come thru Miami, where many of them stay.

MTT: During an interview with the CEO of Jackson Memorial International, he reported that they attract 2,500 patients a year internationally — mostly from the Caribbean.
SB: Through Atlanta?

MTT: No, into Miami. There's also interest among Europeans for traveling here.
SB: We are intrigued by oncology innovation in Europe and by the interest Europeans have shown in the United States for quality care. It's likely that we would deepen our market analysis before making any plans. We have a pretty reasonable and effective array of strategic filters that we apply as we look at major decisions.

MTT: Would an offshore hospital allow you to perform procedures and treatments that are not yet FDA-approved — HIFU? Stem cell? Drugs? People are traveling to access care not available in the United States.
SB: Theoretically, we sure could, and our instinct is also to break down the barriers to providing those types of therapies to patients in the USA.

We helped pioneer the creation of the FDA "compassionate use" exception. If you're not familiar with this, it gives caregiver the ability to go to the FDA with a promising therapy and get a one-time exception on an accelerated basis to help a patient who has no other options. Our government needs our help to enhance quality and speed of care, and to keep healthcare in the United States at the forefront internationally.

MTT: Tell us more.
SB: The FDA needs to keep up with rapid innovations in healthcare. At the Center for Health Transformation meeting, we discussed how slow the FDA bureaucracy can be, and how its structure doesn't consider therapies that are being developed in the world of technology and economics. I don't mean to approve new therapies. They aren't even sure who to contact to review innovations with the FDA.

MTT: Can you share information about your revenues?
SB: We're privately held, and still owned entirely by our founder and his family. We don't publish our financials.

I can assure our key audiences that we are growing, financially sound and confident that as long as we provide great care and a wonderful experience, markets will reward us appropriately.

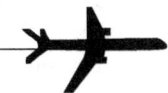

I. Glenn Cohen
Assistant Professor, Co-Director
Harvard Law School
Petrie-Flom Center for Health Law Policy
Biotechnology and Bioethics

May 2011

Glenn Cohen is an Assistant Professor at Harvard Law School and Co-Director of the Petrie-Flom Center for Health Law Policy, Biotechnology, and Bioethics at Harvard Law School. Prof. Cohen is one of the world's leading experts on the intersection of bioethics (sometimes also called "medical ethics") and the law, as well as health law. He also teaches civil procedure. From Seoul to Krakow to Vancouver, Professor Cohen has spoken at legal, medical, and industry conferences around the world and his work has been covered on PBS, NPR, in the Boston Globe, and several other media venues.

Prof. Cohen's current projects relate to reproduction/reproductive technology and to medical tourism – the travel of patients who are residents of one country, the "home country," to another country, the "destination country," for medical treatment. His past work has included projects on end of life decision-making, FDA regulation, research ethics, and commodification.

His award-winning academic work has appeared in the journals such as the Stanford, Southern California, Minnesota, Iowa, and Hastings Law Reviews, the Harvard Journal of Law and Negotiation, the Harvard Journal of Law and Technology, the Food and Drug Law Journal, the Journal of Law, Medicine, and Ethics and the Hastings Center Report.

Prior to joining the faculty, Prof. Cohen served as a clerk to Chief Judge Michael Boudin, U.S. Court of Appeals for the First Circuit. He also served as an appellate attorney for the U.S. Department of Justice, Civil Division, Appellate staff, where he acted as lead counsel in over 12 Circuit Court cases and represented the United States in the U.S. Supreme Court, in conjunction with the Solicitor General's office. Immediately before joining the faculty he was a fellow at the Petrie-Flom Center.

Prof. Cohen has published two papers on medical tourism, with two additional papers soon to be published and several more on the way. The two published papers are:
- *Protecting Patients with Passports: Medical Tourism, Medical Tourism and the Patient-Protective Argument*, 95 Iowa Law Review 1467 (2010). Available for free download at: http://ssrn.com/abstract=1523701
- *Medical Tourism: The View from 10,000 Feet*, 40 Hastings Center Report, March- April, 11 (2010). Available for free download at: http://ssrn.com/abstract=1650616

***Medical Travel Today* (MTT): From a legal perspective, how would you divide the medical travel landscape?**
Glenn Cohen (GC): I think of medical tourism as coming in three flavors. The first is medical tourism for services that are legal in the home country.

The second category is medical tourism for services that are legal in the destination but not the home country. This is what I call circumvention tourism – from abortion tourism and assisted suicide tourism to stem cell therapy tourism and another major market at the moment, reproductive technology access tourism.

The third category is medical tourism for services that are illegal in both the destination and the home country, for example organ sale tourism. It's also helpful to divide between three types of patient populations, based upon how they are accessing care.

The first example is the patient paying out-of-pocket, which includes the uninsured and underinsured in the U.S. The second is the privately insured medical tourism patient, which I think is growing.

And the third category – which admittedly has not yet really taken off in the U.S. -- is the government-prompted medical tourism. This isn't completely new, since there has been a (failed) attempt by West Virginia to get their public employees to use medical tourism, and proposals from Medicare and Medicaid here in the U.S. to lay the groundwork.

Where medical tourism is legal in both the home and destination country, we've got patient protection concerns which relate to the quality of care in the destination facilities, as well as the quality of follow up care.

We've got some problems that are becoming more familiar: Basically, the difficulty in recovering damages from medical malpractice for U.S. patients who go abroad. We also have referral liability for doctors in the US or other home countries that refer patients.

There are also dynamic effects on prices and regulatory status in the U.S. So with enough competition, there's suddenly pressure for a race to the top or bottom, pressure for regulation and price pressure in terms of doctors fees.

MTT: How can US physicians who provide follow up care for medical travelers protect themselves against a lawsuit?
GC: Great question. There are a couple of ways. First of all, when physicians treat patients prior to the patient traveling abroad, the physician is connected to the patient.

Let's begin by talking about the referral situation. There's not a lot of case law on referral liability for international medical tourism. I actually think there may be no case law, at all.

There is, however, robust case law in the U.S. about what the doctor's liability is regarding domestic referrals. I'd like to address some of ways that doctors can avoid making a negligent domestic referral.

Basically, there's some duty of inquiry here. Here are the kinds of cases that we have seen in this area of negligent domestic referrals (not medical tourism) and things that doctors need to avoid: Referring to a doctor that you know is incompetent, a doctor who you know has dementia – or, for example, a doctor who you have a reason to believe or didn't make an inquiry as to whether he or she is licensed in the jurisdiction that they are in.

Again, we don't have any case law in the international arena as to what counts as negligence. But here's some general guidelines for physicians making a referral: One good place to start is to determine whether or not the doctor to whom you are referring is licensed in the jurisdiction being referred to. Also, determine if the facilities are accredited. If a physician gets sued, that would be the kind of thing that would be put into evidence to avoid a claim of negligent referral.

MTT: Do you think that doctors are referring patients abroad?

GC: It depends. There's a formal type of referral, like sending someone to a specialist, and I don't see a lot of that happening. Again, with increasing amounts of insurance policies for medical tourism those referrals are probably going to become more prominent.

Occasionally, what I do see -- although not that often -- is a bit of a soft referral, especially for an indigent patient. I'm not a doctor and I don't see these patients, but I've been told by my doctor friends that have some medical tourism in their practices that this scenario may unfold: The doctor will go over the options and the patient will say they don't have any insurance or resources to pay for the care, and they really can't proceed.

And the patient will say they've heard about medical tourism, and what does the doctor know about it? This may be a kind of soft referral, and it's unclear how the law will treat this. It remains to be seen if this will be treated the same way as hard referrals that we currently have in the U.S. system.

But even if the doctor didn't do a referral at all, if patients are coming back to them for follow up care, I tell doctors they are at an increased risk of getting sued if something has gone wrong. Theoretically, the medical malpractice system is supposed to parcel out the injury, to determine whether the home country physician's error is the cause of an injury versus whether injury was caused by the foreign physician.

When patients have a reduced chance of medical malpractice recovery against the foreign facility, they are more likely to sue the home destination doctor -- if they are going to sue anyone. Although it is theoretically possible that after a trial, the court or the jury will correctly carve out who did what to whom and caused what injury, the home country doctor wouldn't want to be in that situation of having to rely on the court system to make that determination.

Moreover, for medical malpractice insurance, the referring physician may be pressured to settle the case. Before it even gets to that level, I tell physicians that they should think long and hard as to whether they are going to treat patients who want follow up care after receiving treatment at a foreign facility. They should also apply extra rigor in documenting the health care status of the patient who returns to their practice for follow up care. Clearly, these physicians are at increased risk.

All that said, there is also liability in the U.S. for terminating an existing treatment relationship improperly And there are duties incumbent upon providers when there exists a relationship with the patient who comes into your care, although this varies a little bit state by state.

MTT: What is the proper way?

GC: It varies state by state. The cases suggest that while a physician can withdraw from a treatment relationship, he or she must give the patient sufficient notice of the intention to withdraw that the patient can procure other medical attention if desired. The usual practice is for a physician terminating a relationship to find a substitute physician or secure a transfer of the patient to another facility's care, so there is little case law on whether merely providing notice (rather than actually finding a substitute) is enough to avoid liability.

There are also some other relevant rules. It's improper to end a treatment relationship on a certain basis, such as if a person converts to a different religion and you say you don't really treat people of that religion. That would probably violate parts of the civil rights laws.

One thing doctors should consider is how to proceed when a new patient is going to go abroad for treatment. Doctors are ordinarily under no obligation to begin a treatment relationship with a patient. So, if a patient comes to the physician and says, "I think you do medical tourism, and will you provide me with follow up care?" you need to be careful about it.

If you haven't started a relationship, the duties I mentioned don't attach to you. But even if the duties do attach to you, when starting a treatment relationship, it's worthwhile to think about whether you are going to be willing to deal with the patient for follow up. If not, it may be advisable to sort of tell the patient right at that point, not after they've gone abroad and come back for your care.

I don't want to alarm doctors because I'm not aware of any case that's gone to judgment or has resulted in an opinion involving medical tourism. It's hard to know whether that means there have been very few lawsuits or that they have all settled.

MTT: Is there any impact upon a physician's malpractice insurance?
GC: It's good for doctors to treat patients, and it's good for doctors to provide follow up care. But these are a series of things that doctors should think about ahead of time.

They should also talk to their domestic medical malpractice insurer to determine whether and under what circumstance the domestic medical malpractice insurer will cover them for injuries associated with that follow up care or for any suits that involve medical tourism.

It is possible that the terms of the insurance coverage won't cover it. I don't know the details of individual policies. But it's the kind of thing that would be worthwhile to have a conversation about with the insurer before dealing with a patient who is thinking of using medical tourism and wants his or her home doctor to provide follow up care.

MTT: You've addressed patients traveling abroad. What about the growing number of patients traveling to another part of the U.S.?
GC: I call that intra-national medical tourism as opposed to international medical travel tourism. There's definitely some of it going on, and during the last healthcare reform debate, there was a lot of push towards trying to liberate health insurance, make it more intra-national and more portable from state to state.There are a series of ways in which it's similar and yet different from international medical tourism, and it may be useful to look through that.

In terms of a patient seeking medical malpractice liability, the chances of successfully suing the foreign provider are much greater when the provider is another U.S. state than in a foreign. The patient may have to give the case to a lawyer who is licensed in that jurisdiction -- but it's not like finding a lawyer that would be willing to bring your medical malpractice suit in India!

Additionally, the substance of medical malpractice laws varies between states, including things like damage caps loss allocation rules, etc, Ronen Avraham has a good article on the subject entitled "An Empirical Study of the Impact of Tort Reforms on Medical Malpractice Settlement Payments", 36 Journal of Legal Studies S183. I discuss these in my Iowa Law Review paper mentioned above as well

MTT: Can you elaborate?
GC: Between 1980 and 2005, several differences emerged between different states. One example is called "doctrine of joint and several liabilities for medical malprac-

tice." This is where you go after every person -- the hospital or the doctor -- for the full amount or for part of the amount, you have discretion.

There is also the "collateral source rule," which is when you have insurance that covers your damages after the fact. For example, let's say you have health care needs that are going to be paid for from a collateral source -- can you still go after the doctor for that? It's called the collateral source rule.

There is also the circumstance allowing for periodic payments of some amount to cover the damages. Defendants purchase annuities for these payments to relieve themselves of the obligation for paying the patient should the patient die before the periodic payments are exhausted.

Then there are situations where caps have been put on non-economic damages, and in some states, there have been caps on punitive damages.

Finally, there are instances where there have been changes in the evidentiary showing required to receive punitive damages.

On top of all this, there are also differences between how the standard of care is defined at the local level compared to national standards of care. Some states still actually vary on that.

So, there are a number of ways -- roughly speaking, eight or nine dimensions -- by which states formally vary in terms of the law that they apply in medical malpractice. That being said, even within those variations, U.S. states are likely to be more similar in terms of the medical malpractice law than in places like India or Malaysia, for example, where the medical malpractice law is much less patient-friendly.

As I discuss in more depth in my Iowa Law Review paper, for example, Thai laws limit medical malpractice awards and do not compensate for pain and suffering. In India medical negligence claims are rare and multimillion dollar awards are nonexistent. One author claims that while medical malpractice relief is technically available in India, around 95% of cases are dismissed, and the substantial backlog of cases means that the patient may face a lengthy delay before any adjudication, and given the minimal amount of damages likely to be recoverable, the amount of litigation expenses may total more than any potential recovery, making the suit not economically viable.

Some criticize Malaysian and Singaporean med-mal law as doctrinally too deferential to physicians in determining the standard of care and whether that standard was breached in a each case and one author has suggested that Mexican courts do not provide any real recourse to victims of medical malpractice.

One could more easily file a suit in a second U.S. state, and will be able to enforce a judgment against the assets in that state. We have what is called "full faith and credit," where the individual gets a judgment in one U.S. state; and if there's personal jurisdiction, you can take that judgment and bring that over to another state to enforce that judgment. That's not necessarily true in the international context.

The other thing to consider is that we have a huge disparity on the quality side within the U.S.. People who study healthcare quality show that there's significant disparity among different facilities. But the disparity tends to be geographic and not necessarily tied directly to state by state benchmarks. So, in a particular state, you'll have hospitals that are very good and you'll have hospitals that are not nearly as good. In many U.S. states you have much better available information on quality than you do on the international level.

As I said recently at a medical travel conference in Korea, and as I document in my Iowa Law Review paper, people don't use this information too much in the U.S.

context. They tend to rely on friends and anecdotes, not data. But in many of the states like NY, PA and MA, there is some data to go on.

MTT: Do you think this is a time bomb that's ticking away? Is there likely to be case law or any case examples of malpractice in the international marketplace to test what is going on?

GC: Yes, I mean it will happen eventually. The U.S. patient faces a lot of obstacles to collecting damages from a foreign provider. But, there are some things that foreign providers are doing that will make it more likely they will be suable in the U.S.

Let me give you an example I was told about during a recent hospital tour in South Korea. One of the hospitals has a nurse affiliated with a hospital in New York, and is ready to do initial screenings on patients in the U.S. I think that's the kind of relationship that's more likely to subject the foreign provider to jurisdiction in the U.S.

It is the kind of thing that they are doing in the U.S. Chances are, one of these providers will be doing something like that and will be subject to U.S. jurisdiction in court. Then there will be the question of whether the hospital can get the case dismissed on another ground-- either there's no merit to it or it will come under the doctrine known as froum non conveniens, which basically asks the court to dismiss the case because this is not a convenient place to hold a trial – the evidence is elsewhere, among other things.

Eventually, I think we're going to get a case where, in fact, a suit will be maintained in the U.S. and makes it to trial and a judgment. When cases get that far along, the hospital has a large incentive to settle, but if they don't, I think we will eventually get a case that holds a foreign provider liable.

My own guess is that the actual case law that develops won't be all that different from what we hae domestically. It will probably apply to foreign law, but it won't be that different from the way things are analyzed.

Let me take a step back, in terms of a procedure and the way things develop and are maintained in the U.S. courts regarding applying foreign law. It seems unlikely that there will be a lot of the tortious activity actually occurring in the U.S., so as I discuss in my Iowa Law Review article under choice of law principles you'll likely have a U.S. court applying Thai law or Indian Law, or Korean Law in the U.S. court. And the patient may in the end win, and there will be a judgment against a foreign provider. I think that's likely to occur at some point.

MTT: In that case, how likely do you think it would be that the patient would actually collect?

GC: There would be a number of factors. One would be if the foreign facility, after losing at that point, would have a strong incentive not to make the collection difficult.

I think the facility may have a strong public relations reason to want to pay up. The other thing is that in order to get personal jurisdiction in the U.S., it's likely that the foreign facility is doing something in the U.S. so they'll have like an office or something like that. If that's the case, it's possible that the court will attach those assets to satisfy the judgment.

So if you're running a little office where you have a nurse in the U.S., it may be that you attach the furniture or the computers or whatever to satisfy the judgment. My guess is that if a case gets that far along, foreign providers have an incentive to try and get the case dismissed and everything up until that stage.

But once it gets up to that stage -- just for PR reasons alone --they're probably not going to want to fight too hard on the collection. But I don't know. It probably depends upon the size of the foreign provider and how much business they want to do going forward.

I will say that in California, the state thought this through ahead of time. It has authorized some Mexican-based HMOs to sell some insurance plans providing services in Mexico, but in return has required the insurers to consent to personal jurisdiction in the U.S. They must also continuously review the quality of Mexican providers and publish an advisory statement on healthcare in Mexico among other things.

As I discuss in more depth in my Iowa Law Review article, if a U.S. state wants to get ahead of this and is worried, they could require that foreign providers consent to jurisdiction in the U.S. -- or at least consent to arbitration and also make available how a judgment can be collected.

If we're worried about this, each U.S. state or the U.S. federal government can get ahead of this problem and try to solve it before it actually occurs.

MTT: Are you referring to a California HMO that offers coverage in the Baja?
GC: This is actually the opposite. These are Mexican based HMO's. For the California-based HMO's Baja coverage, it's easy in the sense that they are California-based and if there's going to be jurisdiction over them in California, they've got a lot of assets in California.

California initiated this program in 1998, but then expended it in 2004. They basically allowed Mexican-based HMO's to sell insurance plans providing services in Mexico. At the outset, it was only to Mexican nationals living in CA, and then to non-Mexican citizens later on in 2004, although that expansion technically expired in 2008, so I am not sure what the current status is.

But in order for these Mexican-based HMO's to have the privilege of selling insurance products in California, the government pulled them aside and said, "Listen, if you are going to provide services to Californian patients, you must subject yourself to jurisdiction in the California courts. At the end of the day you can't say, I'm sorry – you can't sue me for whatever goes wrong.

So, they gave with one hand, and then they needed this authorization to allow the Mexican-based HMO's to sell products to US patients. In order to do that, they got a concession from them that they would basically consent to jurisdiction in CA.

MTT: How does this differ from the accidental medical tourist who happens to be touring in France or Spain or anywhere in the world and needs medical care -- and it's botched. Does that differ from the patient who intentionally travels for medical care?
GC: It does in a few ways. One way is in terms of the patient who travels to France and gets botched there. The chance of recovery in the US is even less, unless they happen to go to a facility that has a huge presence -- like the sister organization of an American facility.

Usually we call this "specific in personam personal jurisdiction," which means that normally jurisdiction has to be predicated upon a tie that has to be related to the thing you're suing about. So in the case of the regular medical tourist, there are possible ties in that the foreign provider advertising/recruiting in the U.S.—sort of reaching into the U.S. is the image.

In the kind of case you're talking about, where you just happen to have a foreign facility just sitting there, it may not have any ties to the U.S. Even if it does have ties, they tend to be unrelated to the actual touring that occurred, because it's not like they did anything that brought this patient to them.

So, in that case, the accidental tourist is going to have a harder time suing in the U.S. than the active intentional medical tourist, assuming that the foreign provider in that case has made some attempt to reach out to this patient.

MTT: Since the U.S. is a major destination for medical tourism – I think it is rated in the top three destinations -- do foreigners have rights to sue the hospitals and providers here if the case is botched?
GC: Absolutely. They can absolutely bring suit in the U.S.

MTT: Do they?
GC: I've seen a few cases here and there involving foreign patients who've sued in the U.S. I haven't seen a lot, but this is something that I have not systematically reviewed, so I cannot speak authoritatively on that.

Certainly, they have a lot of incentive to do so because the U.S. law tends to be more remunerative than most of their home state laws, and our jury and discovery rules are also very attractive. If there are going to sue anywhere, it's a good idea to sue in the U.S., all things being equal.   We are on the generous end in terms of medical malpractice.

MTT: Would they likely hire a U.S.-based attorney?
GC: Yes. I would think it advisable to have somebody here that is well experienced at medical malpractice in that particular state.

MTT: Are there any additional words of advice that you would give to our readers?
GC: One thing that I would think about might be how the Affordable Care Act (the Obama health reform) is going to change the dynamics of the market for them – that might be interesting.

What I usually tell people is that while the number of uninsured individuals is going to decrease, it's not going to go completely away, even if the Act is completely implemented in 2019. The Congressional Budget Office estimated that there would be about 23 million non-elderly that will still be uninsured. Of those, many of them – about one third -- will be undocumented aliens and many of them will be from Mexico.

In the uninsured market, I think you'll see a decrease in the total size of the market and an increase in the number of people who are going to Mexico -- that tends to be a favorite destination for undocumented individuals from that region.

The uninsured market is going to contract, but it is unclear as to the size of the underinsured market. It will likely depend a little bit upon how good one's insurance has to be to satisfy the Secretary of Health and Human Services in terms of the mandate. It's possible it will stay the same or it's possible that it will actually grow a little bit if the plans that come into existence because of the mandate are actually leaving a lot of people underinsured.

I also think the insured market is likely to increase because now there will be much more demand for lower cost insurance products. It's possible that the HHS Secretary will use her discretion -- she has been delegated a lot of discretion to determine what kind of a plan will satisfy the insurance mandate.

Theoretically, she could use that discretion in a way that rules out insurer prompted medical tourism plans. Thus far, however, she hasn't shown any inclination to do so, as far as I am aware of. I do think there's a chance that the medical travel market will increase.

One last note for your readers is that there is no case law on how facilitators are going to be treated for medical malpractice purposes. But as I discuss in the Iowa Law Review paper, there's a chance that they are going to be treated under a more friendly status than the HMO's which get into medical malpractice lawsuits.

I expect that facilitators will be better off in terms of the substance of medical malpractice law that they face. On the other hand, facilitators are much more likely to be subject to jurisdiction in federal courts and have suits maintained against them in federal courts, because they have many more contacts with the U.S. So I do think there's a difference that cuts both ways. On one hand, there are more likely to be lawsuits against facilitators than physicians in foreign facilities. On the other hand, they're more likely to be judged by a more favorable standard than the foreign doctors and foreign facilities.

MTT: Do you put travel agents into that bucket?
GC: Probably not.

A travel agent who operates in the U.S. is likely to be subject to a lawsuit in the U.S., that much is clear. But whether they're going to be sue-able on the medical malpractice theory depends, I think, a little bit on how they hold themselves out and what they actually do.

If you're just looking to arrange travel for a patient to go abroad and harm results not from the travel but from the delivery medical services abroad, I would think it would be hard to get a successful lawsuit against you.

On the other hand, if you are behaving like a facilitator – brokering, arranging and handling the back-and-forth with the foreign hospital -- then I think you're more likely to be subject to potential liability.

MTT: If you're an illegal alien and you access care in the U.S., do you have rights to sue for malpractice?
GC: As far as I know, the answer is yes.

The fact that you're illegal alien, you haven't given up your medical malpractice liability rights – just as if someone ran you over by a car or a toaster exploded. Just because you are an undocumented alien, you wouldn't lose your rights.

Now, you might have a strong incentive not to bring a lawsuit because of course, bringing the lawsuit your undocumented status would be revealed. But there's nothing that prevents you from bringing the lawsuit. And the last thing I am going to say is about people getting insurance business here. As I mentioned before, California has adopted this kind of authorizing regime. Texas has adopted the opposite regime, basically prohibiting insurance with medical tourism products. It seems as though the intention of the statute was to actually block off insurer-prompted medical tourism completely, but it was not clear if that was worded correctly to do that and it may just block insurance products that require some amount of medical tourism – I discuss this issue in my Iowa Law Review piece.

Through their existing HMO and Preferred Provider Organization (PPO) statutes, many states already have indirectly regulated medical tourism, making insurer prompted medical tourism programs more difficult to implement. The exception is self-insured companies.

Companies that self insure are not governed by the state HMO or PPO regulations, due to what's called ERISA-preemption. That's one of the reasons we've seen the most interest and growth thus far in the self-insured market. But it's possible to conclude that if insurers are interested in a bigger share of the pie – meaning that in many states 40-60 percent of the patients are already covered by a self-insured plan -- that's a pretty big slice of the pie.

If Insurers are interested in yet a bigger slice of the pie, they can always seek to get an exemption from the PPO or HMO statute as it applies to medical tourism. Or, they can try to get the state to implement something like what California has done, which sort of authorizes insurer-prompted medical tourism.

It's sort of worthwhile for them to think about it both ways, in which the existing regulation may block them accidentally and the way in which it may be possible to induce a state government to try and change its regulation of medical tourism. It just is not on the radar of most state governments outside of TX and CA. Most states haven't really thought it through.

CRUDE! A Story of Passion in Aruba

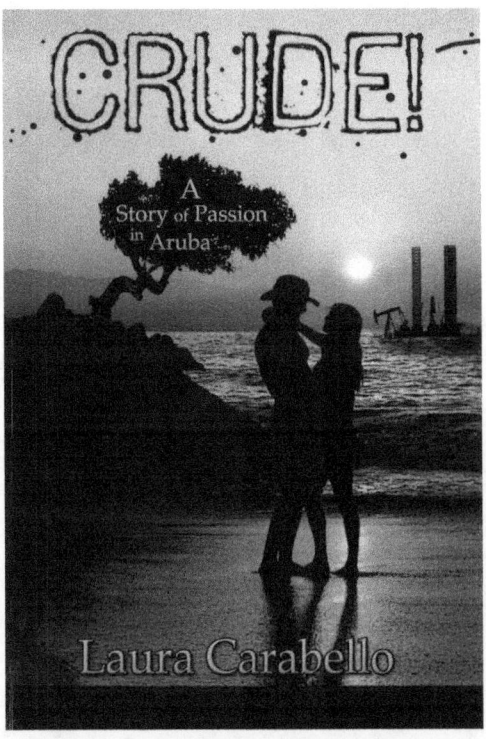

Debra Sheffield dies with a dark secret. A gold locket containing a time-worn photo of a man with an inscription in an unfamiliar language leads her daughter Maggie on a tumultuous search for the truth. *CRUDE! A Story of Passion in Aruba* recounts Debra's life and her stormy marriage to Mike Sheffield—the handsome, wealthy business executive who becomes chairman of the world's leading oil production and refinery company. Their high-profile life sweeps them to Aruba, a largely undiscovered island in the Caribbean during the 1960s. Life is anything but serene in this tropical paradise. Restless and unable to conceive, Debra resents everything—including her husband. She indulges in an illicit, passionate affair with a local Afro-Aruban and becomes pregnant...unsure of who the child's biological father is. Throughout her life, Debra never reveals her suspicions to anyone. Four decades later, the mystery unravels in modern day Aruba where Maggie searches for her true identity.

Paperback, 417 pages
6" x 9"
ISBN 1-4241-2650-9